Fundamentals of the Speech and Language Sciences

....

Fundamentals of
the Speech and
Language Sciences

....

William R. Culbertson, PhD
Professor, Communication Sciences and Disorders
Northern Arizona University
Flagstaff, Arizona

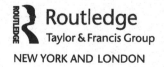

Routledge
Taylor & Francis Group

NEW YORK AND LONDON

Cover Artist: Justin Dalton

First published in 2020 by SLACK Incorporated

Published in 2024 by Routledge
605 Third Avenue, New York, NY 10158

and by Routledge
4 Park Square, Milton Park, Abingdon, Oxon, OX14 4RN

Routledge is an imprint of the Taylor & Francis Group, an informa business

© 2020 Taylor & Francis Group

Library of Congress Control Number:2019941971

ISBN: 9781630913489 (pbk)
ISBN: 9781003524298 (ebk)

DOI: 10.4324/9781003524298

Dedication

This book is dedicated to my editor and wife (not necessarily in that order), Kristan E. Culbertson. Special thanks are extended to Mathew DeVore, who prepared some of the figures for this book.

Contents

Dedication ....*v*

Introduction ....*ix*

Chapter 1   The Scientific Method 1

Chapter 2   Basic Physics 7

Chapter 3   Basic Acoustics 17

Chapter 4   Introduction to Acoustic and Articulatory Phonetics 37

Chapter 5   Neuroscience of Speech and Language 49
            Part 1: Speech Production and Perception 49
            Part 2: Cortical Centers for Language Production and Perception 57
            Part 3: Motor Functions of the Central Nervous System 68
            Part 4: Listening 73

Chapter 6   Speech Systems 79
            Part 1: Respiration and Speech 79
            Part 2: Phonation and Speech 87
            Part 3: Articulation and Speech 93

Introduction

Welcome to the world of discovery in speech and language sciences.

This book addresses the fundamentals of the speech and languages sciences. As such, the content is a general exploration, at a fundamental level, of acoustics, respiratory science, voice production and science, acoustic phonetics, and speech sound spectrography and instrumentation. Language representation and motor programming as they pertain to the dynamic process of speech communication are also explored, as are the fundamentals of speech perception.

Look for interesting figures containing historical information about seminal scientists and scholars who contributed to the topics under discussion.

This publication will be of interest to undergraduate students in communication sciences and disorders programs, and may also be of interest to students in music (voice), special education, and speech communication. Graduate students in communication sciences and disorders may also find this work a helpful refresher.

—William R. Culbertson

The Scientific Method

GOAL

Examine how knowledge is acquired, with a focus on scientific knowledge and the scientific method.

OBJECTIVES

○ Distinguish the scientific method from other means of acquiring knowledge.
○ Examine hypothesis testing as a means of inferring knowledge.
○ Distinguish dependent variables from independent variables.
○ Distinguish among the four major parts of a scientific research paper.

• • • • • •

ACQUIRING KNOWLEDGE

If we are to study speech sciences, we should first examine the concept of science and how knowledge is gathered. Sometimes a friend comes up with the comment such as, "They have proven such-and-such a fact." Who are "They" anyway? Shouldn't we have a notion of what processes led to their conclusions? Obviously, the best way to answer those questions is to read the relevant study report for ourselves. And as we do read the report, whether it is focused on speech and language or on other scientific matters, why should we believe, or how much of what we read should we believe? A discussion of scientific thinking will help us put these matters in perspective.

Briefly put, scientific thought is the result of humankind's attempts to understand and, to the extent possible, control the universe. Human beings have developed various means by which to manage their universe. These include ritualistic ceremonies, with differing degrees of success. However, over the millennia, one

Culbertson, W. R.
Fundamentals of the Speech and Language Sciences (pp 1-6).
© 2020 Taylor & Francis Group.

relatively reliable method has evolved, and that is the *scientific method*.

Going back to the earliest people, at a time when human brains were just beginning to show signs of thought, we might imagine that one of the first things the ancient people observed was that some things happened without their direct participation, and that other circumstances appeared to be the result of some action.

Ancient human beings must have noticed that they had nothing to do with some things happening. For example, plants, some edible and some not, sprang from the earth without any intervention from human beings. The causes were unknown, and attributed, we know, to supernatural beings such as gods or aliens or the like. At some point, earliest people may have figured out that some of their actions, conscious or not, had results, and finally concluded that there was a cause-effect relationship between their actions and results. In other words, the ancient people discovered that they could reliably cause changes in their world by performing certain actions.

To extend our illustration, someone or some group of people must have, at some point, identified seeds and began to cultivate them to the benefit of the individual and the group. As time went on, people found that they could modify their planting processes, or add substances to the soil or adjust the amount of water to supply, and the results were more or healthier plant yields. Maybe this is how the science of agriculture began, along with a series of trials that continue to this day. Other ancient people may have noticed that when two certain kinds of rocks struck each other, sparks were created, and after much early scientific experimentation, the field of heating, ventilation, and air conditioning was created.

In any event, conclusions that our actions have results can only be described as assumptions until there is enough evidence to establish a cause-effect relationship beyond a reasonable doubt. All assumptions are subject to change as more information becomes forthcoming, usually as the result of asking more precise questions or by asking the same questions repeatedly to see if the answers are reliable. Even then, one would be wise to remain a little skeptical. This assertion applies to speech, language, and hearing sciences, as well any other branch of human discovery.

As the quest for more valid and reliable information continued, human beings began to count and measure the relationships among objects, events, causes, and effects. We still do this. We call actions objects, and effects *variables*, and we measure them with *parameters*.

Our explanations of the relationships among parameters, actions, and events are called *theories*.

SCIENTIFIC KNOWLEDGE

Different kinds of knowledge are available to humankind. The kind of knowledge we are interested in here is scientific knowledge, but that doesn't mean that other kinds of knowledge aren't available. Examples of other kinds of knowledge are subjective knowledge, intuition, and spiritual convictions. Scientific knowledge is distinguished from other kinds of knowledge by its reliance on *hypothesis testing*.

Most, if not all, of our so-called scientific knowledge today has been gathered gradually, over a long series of careful observation and hypothesis testing. Sometimes, hypothesis testing leads us to conclude that some item of knowledge we had previously accepted as true was somewhat less than true, only true under certain circumstances, or downright false. More often, we gather just a little bit more of a bigger picture.

The quest for scientific knowledge all begins with a question. "How does this happen?" or "Are these things related?" are the kinds of questions that kick off volumes of published research. The hard part seems to be how to ask the question first, then how to go about finding answers for it.

HYPOTHESIS TESTING

Scientific knowledge has developed over the past few centuries in two manners: deduction and induction. Deduction begins by assuming a general principle and then uses it to explain observations. A typical research question to use deductive reasoning might be, "Why do 10-year-old children articulate speech more like adults than 3-year-old children?" Using the general principle that human children develop to become more like adults as they age would provide a basis for the deduction that the speech and hearing mechanisms of young children are immature. Another way to arrive at a scientific conclusion is through induction. Induction seeks to develop a general principle from multiple observations. A good inductive research approach to the same question might be, "Since the 3-year-old children I've seen have child-like speech, can I assume that all of them do?"

Most scientific research is based on inductive reasoning, whereby the researcher observes the results of variable manipulation and seeks to explain results in terms of a general principle or of several alternative principles. After that, one may use deductive reasoning to explain other observations according to the same principle or principles.

RESEARCH HYPOTHESIS

This book is concerned with the current state of scientific knowledge about speech and language. Therefore, we shall now turn away from the philosophy of science and look at the nuts and bolts of research, the research project.

The first matter to treat is the idea of *proof*. In the sense of establishing the certainty of a fact, or of what is true, the concept of truth is never maintained by inductive research. In other words, nothing is proven by a research project. This may be news to some, but accepting this fact makes the whole world of research make much more sense. Instead, any data obtained by collective experiments either add to or fail to support a contention, or are consistent or not consistent with a principle.

Within inductive reasoning, researchers typically begin with an idea to test a hypothesis. This means they begin with a *research hypothesis*.

Here are a few examples of typical research hypotheses, chosen at random from the body of literature in communication and its disorders:

"Bilingual children with language impairment differ from typically developing children in the accuracy of using past tense morphology," (Jacobson & Schwartz, 2005).

" ... if empathy is subserved by gray matter differences, participants with higher scores on affective empathy will have greater gray matter density in the insula whilst individuals who score higher on cognitive empathy will have greater gray matter density in the MCC/dmPFC [mid-cingulate cortex and adjacent dorsomedial prefrontal cortex]," (Eres, Decety, Louis, & Molenberghs, 2015).

"Embryos can discriminate speech sounds," (Eres, Decety, Louis, & Molenberghs, 2015).

" ... children and adults would match auditory speech to the appropriate visual articulation with greater-than-chance accuracy and perform better in AV [auditory-visual] conditions than in auditory only conditions," (Lalonde & Holt, 2015).

After developing a research hypothesis, the researcher then tests it in an experimental design, controlling conditions to the extent possible and manipulating independent variables to see their effects in dependent variables. Fewer variables allow for stronger inferences from the results.

INFER OR IMPLY

Two verbs play important roles in the effective and efficient use of research findings. These verbs, often erroneously taken and used as synonyms, are to *infer* and to *imply*. To infer means to arrive at a conclusion based on observations. To imply means to present behavior or effects with the intention to cause an inference. Thus, when we opine that data or results imply a certain conclusion, what we really mean is that we infer that they do. Inferential statistical methods are designed to help us make inferences, based on observations, with a specified degree of certainty.

When the observations are apparent, the researcher describes these directly, and frequently uses inferential statistical means to determine the probability that the reverse of the experimental hypothesis, called the null hypothesis, can be rejected. That is, researchers posit that the strength of an argument against support of a null hypothesis is an equally strong argument supporting the experimental hypothesis. Then, using inferential statistical means, experimenters express the strength of their argument as percent probability. The percentage is specified by the experimenters and interpreted by readers as a numerical representation of the strength of the experimenters' argument. This is the same as saying, "We're 99.999% sure that we can reject the idea that the opposite of our experimental hypothesis is true."

While this means of deriving research conclusions seems cumbersome at first, a few minutes in consideration of the process reveals it to be elegant and persuasive. It is a far cry from saying, "We have proven our experimental hypothesis," but it makes much more scientific sense. In fact, this approach to investigating scientific questions leaves a 0.001% chance that the null hypothesis is in fact true.

VARIABLES

One very important goal of scientific research is to clarify how the effects of change in one condition may be accompanied by changes in another condition.

For example, a scientific query might wonder how hot the temperature of a metal must be before it melts, or how a clinical stimulus might change the behavior of a patient.

A variable is an entity that changes, and researchers hope that if they can observe enough variable changes, they might be able to tie them together in some way. Here it is important to note that associating a change in one variable with a change in another variable is not the same as inferring that the first change caused the second change.

To better study variable changes, seekers of scientific knowledge distinguish two kinds of variables: the *independent variable* and the *dependent variable*. Independent variables are controlled by the experimenter. These variables are said to be independent because an experimenter is free to assign any quality, value, or magnitude to them. Laboratory conditions, or the physical environment in which the experiment is conducted, are included in this category, since experimenters can manipulate them. Researchers most often seek to stabilize as many independent variables as they can, so they can concentrate on manipulating one or maybe just a few independent variables of greater interest.

Dependent variables change or take on their values as a result of manipulations of the independent variables. Thus, the values of dependent variables may change, or depend, so to speak, on the values of independent variables. The extent to which changes in dependent variables can be logically associated with changes in independent variables is the primary target of an experiment. To get as close as they can to hitting that target, experimenters try to limit the number of independent variables operating in an experimental design. If many independent variables are operating in an experiment, the association of independent variable change with dependent variable change might be less certain.

TYPES OF RESEARCH DESIGNS

Several ways to explore scientific knowledge have emerged to allow more flexibility in scientific observation. These are called *research designs*. Major types of research designs are quantitative research, experimental research, quasi-experimental research, clinical research, and qualitative research.

Quantitative research, as its name implies, is focused on examining quantities through hypothesis testing. The important benefit of using a quantitative research design is control over variables. Such control comes at some cost in flexibility, but the precision resulting from variable control makes it worthwhile to give up some flexibility. A quantitative research design may be parametric, wherein exact measurements or parameters are recorded and reported, or it may be inferential, wherein the observations of small samples are used to infer similar results in a larger group. It is not hard to see that precise control of variables makes inferences more accommodating.

Experimental research is a type of strictly controlled quantitative research. It is distinguished by the establishment of experimental and control groups, to which experimenters randomly assign subjects. Manipulation of independent variables is a fundamental aspect of experimental research, and results are always best explained in terms of the strictly controlled experimental conditions.

Quasi-experimental research is conducted as much like experimental research as possible, but under conditions that strictly adhere to true experimental research designs. In a quasi-experimental research design, it may be impossible or unethical to randomly assign subjects to experimental or control groups, or control of experimental conditions may be beyond the reach of the experimenters. Still, the value of quasi-experimental inferences is not to be ignored.

Clinical research is a special kind of quasi-experimental research or qualitative research. It is carried out to answer treatment questions, and it often involves the use of one or more actual patients in a clinical setting. Clinical research is subject to experimental conditions that are often difficult for experimenters to control. Ethical concerns, such as subject assignments to experimental and control groups, also play a limiting role in clinical research.

Finally, qualitative research is more flexible but less controlled. In cases where variables have multi-faceted, complex interactions and where these interactions are poorly understood, qualitative research designs present a good way to begin examining phenomena as a preparation for future quantitative research. Its advocates use qualitative research designs to study complex phenomena and to arrive at multi-faceted descriptions, but with little attempt to quantify results.

In a very real way, clinical research designs are used regularly by practicing clinicians but rarely published for consumption by the scientific community. When a patient presents a clinical question regarding diagnosis or treatment design, a thoughtful clinician might well design a session to reveal clues to the answer to the question. For example, it might be discovered through clinical research that a pediatric patient produces velar plosives regularly in a back vowel phonetic context than in a front vowel context. Such an inference might be the basis for a modified lesson plan at the next therapy session.

RESEARCH PAPERS

The vast preponderance of research findings is disseminated in research papers, online or on paper. Research papers take on different forms, but most of them have four main parts.

INTRODUCTION AND STATEMENT OF THE PROBLEM

In this section, the research question is presented and explained. This tells the reader about the significance of the study and why it was conducted. It also usually presents the research hypothesis and sometimes a null hypothesis. In very general terms, research hypotheses seek to support differences between groups of subjects. Although they are often implied, rather than stated, one might summarize a typical research hypothesis as follows: "Group AAA is significantly different than group BBB."

Following is an example of a research hypothesis: "Bilingual children with language impairment differ from typically developing children in the accuracy of using past tense morphology," (Jacobson & Schwartz, 2005).

A null version of that research hypothesis would be, "Bilingual children with language impairment do not differ from typically developing children in the accuracy of using past tense morphology." Another expression of the same idea is that there was no difference in the performance of the two groups of children on a certain test of past tense usage. The aim of the experiment is to demonstrate whether or not results support the null hypothesis. The extent to which results fail to support a null hypothesis lend at least tentative support to the experimental hypothesis.

Not all research articles contain an explicit statement of a null or a research hypothesis. Instead, the hypotheses are implied through one or more research questions. Here is an example of a research question: "Is Group AAA significantly different than group BBB?"

REVIEW OF THE LITERATURE

The second section of the standard research paper presents the history of scientific study on the research question. The authors will go back as far as necessary, depending upon the topic, to review what others have done before. This section is important because it provides a foundation upon which to base the present and possibly future studies. It also may explain the present authors' approach to answering the questions.

METHODS

In the third section, authors describe, as closely as possible, the experimental design of their study. Experimental design refers to all concrete factors contributing to how experimenters conducted the study. This includes details about the subjects, how they were selected and how the experimenters organized them into groups, a thorough description of the environment in which subjects are exposed to variable changes, and detailed descriptions of any stimuli presented to subjects.

A proper methods section must also include specifications of any equipment used to manipulate variables and to record results. Such details are also very important as a basis for future research because the strength of conclusions is largely based on the circumstances under which the experimenters observed the results. After all, outcomes of experiments conducted in a hot environment, for example, might differ from those conducted in cold environments.

The value of experimental results to others is influenced by the degree to which experimenters can remain free of bias or of opinions about what they expect outcomes to be. Strong, ethical researchers try to have no expectations about the outcomes of their experiments, no matter what findings they or others have uncovered in the past. Experimenters are interested in the outcomes, whatever they might be, and experimenters should be open to the possibility that outcomes might differ from those reported in previous studies.

RESULTS AND DISCUSSION

In the final section, the authors write of their findings and their inferences about what the findings may mean. In the final section, conclusions must be reasonable based on the experimental design presented in the third section. It is acceptable, often desirable, to present more than one set of possible conclusions derived from the data. Conclusions often form the seeds of suggestions for further study. Replications of experiments are also of value, since results of similar studies with only minor variations may differ in important ways.

LANGUAGE OF THE RESEARCH PROJECT

The language used to describe the gathering of little bits of scientific knowledge is best chosen carefully to support the notion that nothing is proven by a single research project. As we have seen, research projects seek to support or fail to support a null hypothesis. It is most honest to use language that supports the notion that reported events and observations are those that occurred at a given time and were performed by certain experimenters.

First, everything should be written in the past tense. This means that what the researchers observed was simply what happened under those particular conditions at one particular time. Such language implies that if the experimenters had made their observations on another day, things might have turned out differently ... or they might have turned out exactly the same. Further, if they, or somebody else, try the same things at a future time, the result may or may not be the same.

The same principle holds true for clinical report writing. Using the past tense in reports of clinical evaluations or of progress notes presents the facts as they occurred at a specified point in time. Such facts may or may not occur again during a future encounter with a client or patient. For example, instead of reporting that, "Mr. Patient's responses to pure-tone hearing screening stimuli are within normal limits," a more useful and honest statement is, "Mr. Patient's responses to pure-tone hearing screening stimuli were within normal limits." This indicates that Mr. Patient would not need to make an appointment with an audiologist as a result of that screening, but Mr. Patient might need to visit an audiologist at some time in the future.

Second, writers should only use the active voice. Using the active voice, a writer can indicate that the subject of a sentence performed an action upon an object. The subject of a sentence using the passive voice, on the other hand, is the recipient of an action, and the performer of the action need not be identified. Active voice stipulates who manipulated any independent variables. Instead of writing, "The independent variable was manipulated," a more precise, informative and accurate description would be, "Experimenters manipulated the independent variable," to make clear the fact that someone else, such as the subjects themselves, did not manipulate the independent variable.

Once again, this writing principle holds true for clinical report writing. Instead of writing, "Test was administered, and Ms. Patient scored within one standard deviation of the mean," the proper way to write that observation is, "Ms. Patient's responses to Test were within one standard deviation of the mean."

The two linguistic principles, writing active voice and using the past tense, along with the other principles of the research project, are also good ideas for use in clinical as well as research writing—since, in a very real way, clinical writing is a form of research writing. Although it is not often specified as such, clinicians are performing one-subject design clinical research on patients whenever they seek to control clinical conditions, manipulate stimuli they present to patients, and record results as objectively as possible.

REFERENCES

Eres, R., Decety, J., Louis, W. R., & Molenberghs, P. (2015). Individual differences in local gray matter density are associated with differences in affective and cognitive empathy. *Neuroimage, 117,* 305-310.

Jacobson, P. F., & Schwartz, R. G. (2005). English past tense usage in bilingual children with language impairment. *American Journal of Speech-Language Pathology, 14,* 313-323.

Lalonde, K., & Holt, R. F. (2015). Preschoolers benefit from visually salient speech cues. *Journal of Speech-Language-Hearing Research, 58,* 135-150.

Maxwell, D. L., & Satake, E., (2006). Research and Statistical Methods in Communication Sciences and Disorders. Clifton Park, N.Y.: Thomson Delmar Learning.

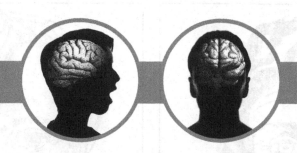

Basic Physics

GOAL

Present basic physical science concepts.

OBJECTIVES

- Distinguish among the three branches of classical physics.
- Identify the branch of physics that studies acoustics.
- Distinguish between fundamental quantities and derived quantities.
- Distinguish among force, mass, acceleration, and their measurement units.
- Distinguish among power, velocity, pressure, and their measurement units.

• • • • • • •

BASIC PHYSICS

The science of physics may be considered as mankind's attempt to quantify, or apply numerical values, to the universe. In physics, the emphasis is on quantities and, of course, quantitative research. Such emphasis on quantities means the physical approach to a description of the universe must be precise in its definitions of, and use of, quantities.

First, a definition of *quantity* is in order. For the present purposes, a quantity is a characteristic of magnitude ("how much") or multitude ("how many").

Some will argue that there are other approaches to study the universe, such as religion, metaphysics, or philosophy. Those approaches and others are equally valid points of view, but in our present study, we adopt the physical approach.

In the earliest times, so little scientific thought had been devoted to the nature of the universe that

Culbertson, W. R.
Fundamentals of the Speech and Language Sciences (pp 7-16).

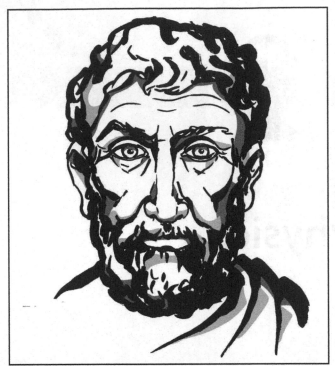

Figure 2-1. Thales of Miletus (a city located in today's western Turkey) is widely regarded as one of the earliest scientists and as one of the seven sages of ancient Greece. Writings of others suggest that he was highly regarded around 600 BCE. Although none of his writings have been discovered in the modern era, he was said to have distinguished himself by proposing scientific ideas without mystical or religious reference, allowing scholarly argument to the contrary. Thales is credited with the notion that the essence of the universe is water, with developing geometric principles through induction, and with setting the yearly calendar for the seasons and equinoxes. (Marusya Chaika/Shutterstock.com)

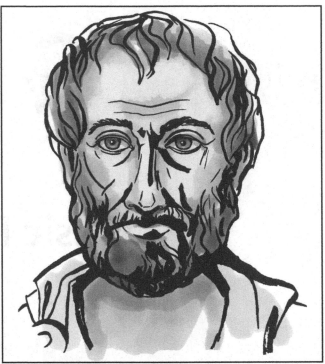

Figure 2-2. Aristotle was born in 384 BCE in Stagira, Greece, and died in 322 BCE Chalcis, Euboea. The scope of his writing is broad, including writings in science, philosophy, politics, and rhetoric. Most of his work is considered antiquated today, but his propositions regarding logical syllogism are essential to modern scientific thought. His understanding of the role of subjectivity in scientific observation remains important, though often neglected. (Marusya Chaika/Shutterstock.com)

chemistry, biology, astronomy, engineering, philosophy, physics, and more could be combined into one science. Ironically, the more we learn about the universe, the closer we are returning to the same situation.

One of the first physical observations was the relationship between the state of water and its temperature. Although none of his original writings have been preserved, the thoughts and studies of Thales of Miletus (see Figure 2-1) were recorded in the writings of other scholars, such as Aristotle. Around 500 years before the common era (BCE), Aristotle (see Figure 2-2) recorded that Thales considered water as no less than the essence of the universe (O'Grady, n.d.).

At around the turn of the 20th century, astounding discoveries in electromagnetism and thermodynamics led to the development of quantum mechanics, and ultimately to the physics of today: modern physics. These discoveries focused on the existence and behavior of the particles that comprise atoms. Before those discoveries, physical science was based on stable frames of reference and on principles held forth for centuries

by the likes of Galileo Galilei (see Figure 2-3) and Isaac Newton (see Figure 2-4).

The discoveries of the modern physics had such far-reaching effects that today physics is often divided into two branches: modern physics and classical (Newtonian) physics. There is only one science of physics, but, for the beginner, the self-imposed limitations of classical physics simplify the study of certain mechanical phenomena. Classical physics relies on the assumptions that the world is three-dimensional, that the frame of reference for observations is inertial (time is not relative), and that mass and energy are conserved. As you may guess, modern physics does not assume a three-dimensional universe. Time, the fourth dimension, is relevant to the frame of reference, and mass can be converted into energy. String theoreticians, extending the frontiers of modern physics, propose up to 36 dimensions, at last count.

To the extent that a basic understanding of classical mechanical forces underlies speech and hearing science, we will begin with the principles of classical physics as they apply to the sounds we hear, and particularly to the sounds of speech.

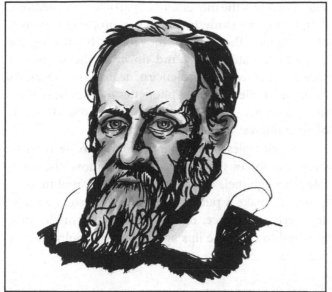

Figure 2-3. Galileo Galilei was born in Pisa, Italy, in 1564 CE and died in Arcetri, Italy, in 1642. He was one of the first to study and posit principles of kinematics, the science of masses in motion. His scientific life was highlighted and impeded by his persecution by the Roman Catholic Church in early 1600 because of his opposition to the heliocentric belief that the earth was the center of the universe. (Marusya Chaika/Shutterstock.com)

MECHANICS, THERMODYNAMICS, AND ELECTROMAGNETISM

Classical physics can be further divided into three large areas: *mechanics*, *thermodynamics*, and *electromagnetism*. Mechanics focuses on movement. Thermodynamics studies the effects of temperature volume and pressure on systems. Electromagnetism studies the characteristics of electromagnetic fields. Intense study of electromagnetism, which had been the object of scientific observation for centuries before 1900 Common Era (CE), served as the trigger for modern physics.

MECHANICS

Mechanics, the study of movement, can be further divided into three branches: *kinematics*, *dynamics*, and *statics*. Kinematics studies trajectories, velocities, and accelerations, without regarding its causes. Kinematic studies can be abstracted to derive algorithms that predict the paths of moving objects, and such objects might include the tongue or other speech articulators. Dynamics is the study of the sources or causes of motion, including forces, pressures, and torques on moving masses. The effects of differing subglottal pressures on vocal fold movements might be a focus of dynamic study. Statics studies physical systems in

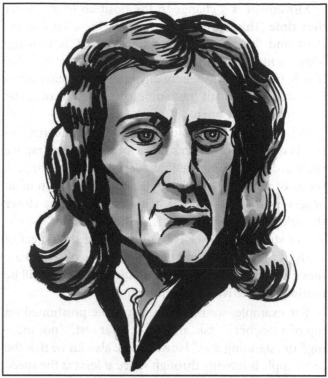

Figure 2-4. Isaac Newton (1643–1727) was one of history's most influential scientists. In 1687, Newton published *Philosophiae Naturalis Principia Mathematica* (*Mathematical Principles of Natural Philosophy*). In that work, Newton presents his three laws of motion, including the second law, from which force equals mass times acceleration is derived. He also discusses the law of inverse squares.

NEWTON'S LAWS of MOTION:
I. Every body perseveres in its state of rest, of uniform motion in a right line, unless it is compelled to change that state by forces impressed thereon.
II. The alteration of motion is ever proportional to the motive force impressed; and is made in the direction of the right line in which that force is impressed.
III. To every action there is always opposed an equal reaction: or the mutual actions of two bodies upon each other are always equal, and directed to contrary parts. (Marusya Chaika/Shutterstock.com)

equilibrium and what properties maintain that equilibrium. Sometimes, an overall system includes subsystems in equilibrium or masses at a constant velocity about the overall system's center of mass. The instantaneous air pressures inside and outside the lungs and intrapleural spaces or the air pressures on either side of the tympanic membrane might be suitable targets for static studies.

The study of masses in motion, a domain of both dynamics and kinematics, is essential to the study of sound, and it takes no great leap of imagination to see how this applies to speech. Dynamics considers masses in terms of *inertia* and *gravitation*. Inertia is the resistance of a mass to a change in its motion state, whether it is moving or at rest. To better understand inertia, the very concept of motion must be explored.

Movement is a change in the position of an object over time. This means if an object is "here" at one instant and "there" at the next instant, it is moving. Movement can be lineal, that is, in a line, or circular, that is, in a circle. Just about any kind of movement can be considered to fall into some combination of lineal and circular movement.

Whether an object is considered to be moving depends upon the observer's frame of reference. First, we must accept the premise that everything is moving. A frame of reference simply applies to the situation of an observer and that which is being observed. The closer the velocity of the observer is to the velocity of the object of study, the lower is the velocity of the object of study. If the observer and the object being observed are moving at the same velocity and direction, they will be motionless relative to one another.

For example, we might see an apple positioned on top of a teacher's desk, and say it is "at rest," "not moving," or "standing still." However, we also know that the same apple is moving through space at least at the speed of the earth's rotation, not to mention at the speed at which the earth orbits the sun, and so on. The apple speed depends upon where the observer is standing. We might see it traveling around 900 miles per hour if we could be in a space station observing the earth's rotation.

Gravitation is a phenomenon also essential to dynamics. It concerns the property whereby masses attract each other. Back in the 17th century, Isaac Newton proposed the theory that all objects, or masses, are attracted to each other by a force. The attraction may be unnoticeable, but it is still there. Anyone who has dropped something is familiar with this force, called *gravity*. Gravity mutually accelerates objects from their current positions to the centers of other objects, and its strength varies with the distances and masses of the objects. The greater the distance between two objects, the weaker the force that creates the acceleration of gravity.

Also, objects having great mass exert greater gravitational force than objects having less mass. According to the theory, that object you dropped is accelerating toward the Earth, just as the Earth is accelerating toward it. Air molecules are attracted to one another in a small way by gravity, although molecular forces exert the most attraction and repulsion between air molecules. Both inertia and gravitation are central to the creation of sound.

Since speech is conveyed by sound energy, an important aspect of speech and hearing science is the study of sound. Acoustics is the study of sound, and, since sound involves the movement of particles in a medium, its quantitative study in physics is properly a branch of mechanics, the study of movement. Narrowing the scope of the study of sound down to the sounds of speech, we arrive at the science of *acoustic phonetics*. As its name implies, acoustic phonetics focuses heavily on the quantitative measurement of speech sounds and is of great interest to speech scientists.

The principles of mechanics may also be used to study the forces that are required to move the vocal folds through their cycles, the amount of amplitude required to make a public address (PA) system audible at a certain distance, or the amount of muscle force required to close the lips against a given pulmonic air pressure.

THERMODYNAMICS

Thermodynamics is the study of temperature, volume, and pressure, and how energy from these sources can be transformed into other forms of energy to perform work. The field expanded greatly in the 19th century as engineers sought to improve the efficiency of steam power as it applied to manufacturing and transportation. Steam power is created by converting the energy contained in liquid water into mechanical energy by heating it until the forces that hold the liquid molecules together are released. Thermodynamic principles also underlie the physiology of pulmonary ventilation and can be applied to the study of respiratory support for speech, as they explain how the flow of air in and out of the lungs is normally accomplished.

Thermodynamic principles are based on four laws, or principles. The first two thermodynamic laws were established in the 19th century, and the third law was formalized in the early 20th century. A fourth law was offered in 1935, but the scientific community felt it to be so fundamental to the first three that it was numbered zero (Fowler & Guggenheim, 1939). Thus, the zeroth law of thermodynamics holds that if two systems are in energy (thermal) equilibrium with a third system, they must be in equilibrium with each other (Fowler & Guggenheim, 1939).

The first law of thermodynamics posits that there is a fixed amount of energy in the universe, and that energy can neither be created nor destroyed. It can, however, change form. For example, energy that is contained, or doing work in a closed system, is called *potential energy*. Potential energy can be imagined as the energy that is contained in a compressed spring, or, for that matter, compressed air. Energy that is acting on elements within or outside of a system, that is, energy that is performing work, is *kinetic energy*. Let that compressed spring go to run a toy, for example, and the potential energy that was stored in that compressed spring is now gradually changing form to become kinetic energy.

Our treatment of thermodynamics would not be complete without mentioning *entropy*. Not all energy in the universe is available to do work. Energy that is not available to do work is measured as entropy and can be imagined as the energy expended in random particle motion. A more concrete example of energy that is not available for work is the random energy lost as heat emanating from the hood of a running automobile engine.

The second law of thermodynamics holds that when two thermodynamic systems are allowed to interact with each other, they will eventually reach a state of entropy or energetic equilibrium with one another. This thermodynamic law is sometimes called Clausius' Law, after Rudolph Clausius (1822 to 1888) (see Figure 2-5). The second law of thermodynamics implies that heat or pressure cannot flow from a region of low amplitude to a region of high amplitude without outside help. This implication is essential to creating the flow of gases during pulmonary ventilation as well as during speech.

The third law of thermodynamics holds that the entropy of an imaginary, completely pure, crystalline system decreases to a constant, potentially zero, as its temperature decreases to absolute zero. At this state, there is theoretically no kinetic motion of the particles that comprise the substance. We would be remiss here if we didn't note that a completely pure crystalline system is an imaginary concept and has thus far never been observed.

ELECTROMAGNETISM

Beginning in the mid-19th century, physicists coalesced what had long been studied concerning electricity. The inclusion of electronic principles with those of classical physics stopped short of quantum physical theories, but included descriptions of electrical potentials in chemical elements, explanations of electrical current flow, and principles of electromagnetic energy waves. Among the fruits of classical electromagnetism were the electric battery, domestic and industrial lighting, motion pictures and television. Quantum physical principles of modern physics involved the electromagnetism of much smaller charges than those studied in classical electromagnetism, such as the charges among subatomic particles within a single atom.

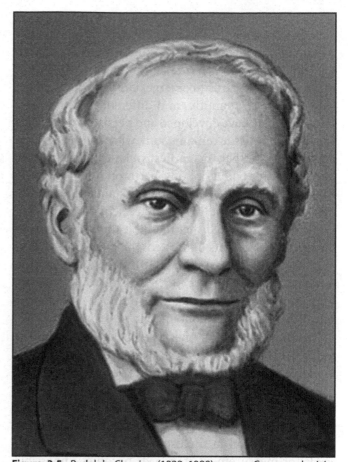

Figure 2-5. Rudolph Clausius (1822–1888) was a German physicist who contributed much to the science of thermodynamics by rewriting or elaborating the first two laws of thermodynamics, which he stated succinctly: "1. The energy of the universe is constant," and, "2. The entropy of the universe aims to approach a maximum." (Clausius, 1865). Clausius thus furthered the evolving concept of thermal entropy and was a major contributor to a kinetic theory of gases, formalized by James Maxwell and Ludwig Boltzman in the 19th century. (Retrieved from http://bre.mkrf.ru/media/2016/10/27/1235197027/15923.jpg)

UNITS, QUANTITIES, AND THEIR RELATIONSHIPS

An essential aspect of physical science is to study the universe in terms of "how many" or "how much." It is therefore essential that physicists have a set of terms or units of measurement to describe all manner of phenomena. Since an important goal of science is to compare physical measurements resulting from various studies, the need for a standard system of measurement units is apparent. Speech and hearing science is one of those phenomena, so a basic understanding of quantities and their units of measurement is in order. The term quantity is used in the study of physics to refer to just such properties of a multitude ("how many?") or magnitude ("how much?").

Throughout history, several measurement systems have been adopted by various cultures. While the existence of a standard set of measuring units is a step in the right direction, it has taken quite some time for a single set of standards to emerge. Unfortunately, different concepts of quantities and different units for their measurements have developed and persisted around the world, and the issue remains somewhat confusing. One might imagine that the earliest measurement systems utilized an individual's body parts or other relatively consistent natural phenomena as standards. Indeed, in a brief history, the U. S. Department of Commerce (NIST, 1974) reported that the Bible and other ancient historical documents indicated that length was first measured with forearm, hand, or finger, and that time was measured by phases of the moon, while volumes were measured by counting the number of stones or certain kinds of seeds contained in vessels.

The most common measurement systems in use today are the metric system, which uses meters, kilograms, and seconds to measure length, mass, and time, respectively, and the British system, which uses feet, pounds, and seconds to measure length, weight and mass, and time, respectively. It should seem obvious that precision in the use of body parts, stones, or seeds for measurement standards becomes impossible because of natural variations between individuals or varying sizes and shapes. Meanwhile, the British system becomes quite unwieldy because different contexts cast different terms for different quantities, such as weight and mass. This leaves the metric system to take preeminence as the most useful standard measurement system. Even the British have converted to the metric system for most quantities, with one notable exception being the use of the pint to measure beer. In the United States, commercial measurement is still done mostly with British system units, while science is usually expressed in metric units.

The most recent iteration of the metric system is contained within a larger system, Le Système International d'Unités, or International System of Units. The International System is often abbreviated, even in English, as SI, for the French Système International. The French designation comes from the fact that the SI was developed in 1971 during an international meeting of physicists in Paris. The official document for the SI standards for U. S. consumption is published by the International Bureau of Weights and Measures (Taylor & Thompson, 2008).

SI is simply an expansion of the widely accepted MKS (meter-kilogram-second) system to add light, heat, molecular quantity, and electric current to the already accepted fundamental quantities of length or distance, mass, and time. This book uses the International System, SI, wherever standard measurements of quantities are required. In general, this means using the meter to measure length, the kilogram to measure mass, and the second to measure time, just as the MKS system did. In cases where the quantities are very small, this text will sometimes follow the lead of speech, hearing, and language sciences convention and revert to the CGS (centimeter-gram-second) system, using the centimeter to measure the length and the gram to measure mass, but always with SI equivalents added.

FUNDAMENTAL QUANTITIES

Quantities are terms that express magnitude and multitude. *Fundamental quantities* are those that cannot be expressed as combinations of other quantities. Rather, fundamental quantities are expressed in terms of their relationships to other fundamental quantities. Whether or not a quantity is considered fundamental depends, at least in part, on the measurement system being used. In SI, the fundamental quantities are length or distance, mass, time, light, heat, molecular quantity and electric current. It is difficult to define fundamental quantities in terms other than their relationships to other fundamental quantities because they are, well, fundamental. Let's have a look at some of the SI fundamental quantities that we will use most: *mass*, *distance*, and *time*. The following definitions of fundamental quantities are given by the *National Institute of Standards and Technology* (NIST), *Special Publication 330*, 2008 Edition (Taylor & Thompson, 2008).

Mass can be defined as the property of an object to resist changes in velocity. Another definition is that mass is the result of dividing force by acceleration. The second definition is based on one of the most basic equations in physics, force is equal to mass times acceleration, or F = MA.

Some people confuse mass with weight. This might well be because they have never left the Earth's gravitational pull, where most masses have weight. Weight, however, is a special kind of force directed toward the center of our planet and other planets by the acceleration caused by gravity. Gravity, the force whereby all masses attract one another, is an inherent property of mass, and increases or decreases with the amount of mass. In other words, if the force of gravity acts with greater effect on a mass, the mass weighs more.

Gravity effects also vary with the proximity of the mass. Thus, masses can be expected to weigh more or less depending upon the planet (or other body) upon which they are found and how close they are to that planet. The gravity of a large planet, such as Jupiter, has a greater effect on NASA's Juno probe than Earth's gravity does at the same distance. If the Juno probe were situated exactly halfway between the two planets, the effect of Jupiter's gravity acting on the probe would be greater than the effect of Earth's, since Earth is the smaller mass.

In SI, mass is measured in kilograms (abbreviated: kg). In November, 2018, the BIPM (French abbreviation: BIPM for Bureau Internationale des Poids et Measures) changed the SI definition of the kilogram from a physical platinum-iridium alloy cylinder known as "Le Grand K," located at the International Bureau of Weights and Measures (BIPM) in Sèvres, France, to a fraction of Planck's constant, ($h = 6.626070150(81) \times 10^{-34}$ J s), a measure relating the energy of a photon to its frequency. According to news stories at the time, the change evoked quite a few emotional responses from some physicists.

Distance, or length, is the one-dimensional measurement of the extension of space between two points. The SI unit of distance or length is the meter (m). It is easy to confuse distance with time since it usually takes an amount of time for a person to travel from one point to another. Often, the answer to the question, "How far is it?" is expressed in time, as in, "Oh, a couple of hours." The SI definition of the meter is the distance light travels in a vacuum over a duration of 1/299,792,458 seconds (Taylor & Thompson, 2008). So in SI, distance is quantified in terms of time.

The SI unit of time is the second (sec). An international standard for a second must be very carefully defined. Time units must be particularly precise because they are essential to functions such as internet timing and global positioning systems that many people depend upon without even knowing it. Even the best clock is far too variable to serve as the basis for such a definition, so some other regularly repeating phenomenon is necessary to set the standard. The International Bureau settled on a form of atomic clock and specified the duration of 9,192,631,770 periods of the transition between two hyperfine levels of the ground state of the cesium 133 atom at zero Kelvin as the definitive second (Taylor & Thompson, 2008).

DERIVED QUANTITIES

Derived quantities, just as the term implies, are those that are the results of manipulating or combining fundamental quantities. For example, velocity is a derived quantity in SI because it is calculated by dividing the distance by time. Some very useful physical quantities are derived, that is, created, through combinations of fundamental quantities. Derived quantities of particular interest for students of speech and hearing sciences include velocity, acceleration, force, volume, density, surface, pressure, work (energy), and power, and their derivations in terms of SI independent units and in terms of SI base units are given in Taylor and Thompson (2008). For this discussion, energy and work are considered equivalent.

VELOCITY

Velocity is distance divided by time, with a directional vector. Velocity is the amount of distance or length (meters) a mass or energy form covers during a given time (in SI, a second) and its direction. The more velocity a mass has, the more distance it can cover in a given time. Simple, isn't it?

Thus, velocity is a quantity derived by dividing the number of meters, or fractions of meters, by the number of seconds, or fractions of seconds, then reducing the fraction down to show how much distance is covered in a single second, always with the direction of travel specified. The SI measure of velocity is created by simply swapping the SI units for distance and time in their proper places: distance ÷ time is meters ÷ seconds. Put another way, velocity is meters/second. Incidentally, whenever a derived quantity is expressed as a result of division or quotient, the division sign (÷) or the slash (/) sign can be said as per. This means velocity can be expressed as meters-per-second.

Some people get velocity and speed confused because both indicate distance covered over time. The difference between these two quantities lies in the fact that velocity is specified in a single direction, while speed is not. If the moving mass changes course during its travel, the original direction, defined in terms of a straight line, still applies, but the time it takes to cover distance in that direction changes. That means velocity changes, too. Imagine hiking toward a mountain lake, but having to go around a large boulder on the way. The direction of your travel would change, slowing your progress (velocity) toward the lake, even though you are walking at the same pace.

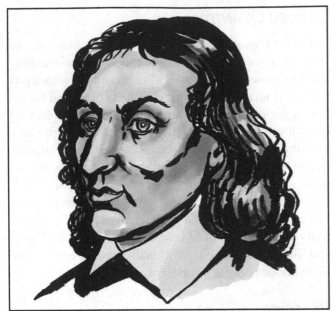

Figure 2-6. Blaise Pascal (1623–1662) was a French mathematician whose work included demonstrations of vacuum principles and led to the creation of the barometer. The SI unit of pressure is the pascal (Pa). (Marusya Chaika/Shutterstock.com)

Speed, on the other hand, has no specified direction. It is still distance divided by time, but with no special direction. Speed is like your pace on the hike to the lake. Even though your direction changed, your pace (speed) did not. The speedometer in an automobile is calibrated to display miles per hour, or distance over time (miles, in the British system, divided by hours, or 360 seconds). Your car, however, can go in just about any direction the road takes, so the gauge on the dashboard is called a speedometer, rather than a velocimeter. Both speed and velocity are calculated with the formula $V = D \div T$.

ACCELERATION

Acceleration is the change in velocity divided by a change in time. It quantifies the rate at which velocity changes, relative to a reference point. Acceleration can be positive or negative, depending upon whether a mass is going faster-and-faster or slower-and-slower. The SI derivation for acceleration is distance divided by time, divided by time. This works out as meters per second per second, or meters $\div$ seconds $\div$ seconds, which is the equivalent of m $\div$ sec $\times$ sec or m $\div$ sec^2.

FORCE

Force is the quantity that changes the acceleration of a mass. This definition applies whether or not the object is already in motion relative to the application of the force. As is the case with velocity, force has both a magnitude, or *scalar* aspect, as well as a directional, or *vector* parameter. That is, force must be described as a number as well as a direction.

In SI, the unit of force is aptly named the Newton (abbreviated N), since Isaac Newton defined it in his second law, very loosely translated and abbreviated as force (F) equals mass (M) times acceleration (A), or $F = MA$. $F = MA$ is one of the most well-known equations in all physics. You may recall that we used that formula when we defined mass as $F \div A$. SI defines a Newton as the amount of force required to accelerate a mass of one kilogram at a rate of one meter per second per second (kg $\times$ m $\div$ sec^2). Specification of force quantities is essential to the study of speech and hearing because the propagation of sound is most commonly the result of applying force to the masses of air molecules.

It is interesting to note that force is a fundamental quantity in the British system, and its unit is the pound. Mass, on the other hand, is a derived ($M = F/A$) quantity in the British system, and the unit of measurement is the slug. Weight is a special kind of force, which, when unopposed, accelerates masses toward the center of the Earth at a rate of approximately 9.8 m/sec^2 in SI units. Note also the relationship between force and time, with force defined in relationship to how much acceleration it imparts to a mass.

PRESSURE, DENSITY, AND VOLUME

It should be apparent that force has little use if it is not applied to mass. If force is applied to a mass, it must, at least, be applied over some portion of the surface of that mass. Surface, in its simplest examples, exists in only two dimensions, and the simplest two-dimensional surface is a square. Sure, other two-dimensional shapes have more sides, and those sides are of various lengths, but we will use the square to begin with to keep matters simple. And, further, the effect of a force on mass below the surface is not of concern at this point, since the layer immediately beneath the surface of two dimensions is just another two-dimensional surface. Therefore, at its simplest, surface is measured as the length (m) of one side of a square multiplied by the length (m) of the adjacent side, or m $\times$ m = m^2. The measure of surface is usually known as area, and abbreviated A.

Pressure is force divided by surface; in SI units, it follows that pressure can be derived as N/m^2. The SI unit for pressure is the pascal (Pa), named in honor of French physicist Blaise Pascal (see Figure 2-6). One pascal is equal to a force of one Newton applied to a surface of one square meter, and the derivation of pressure is $Pa = N/m^2$. The atmosphere around us all has a certain natural pressure. This pressure is measured with a barometer, and meteorologists call this pressure the atmospheric or barometric pressure. It varies widely from time to time, depending upon the weather and the elevation, but the standard reference for barometric pressure is 101.325 Pa. (Taylor & Mohr, 2015). In acoustics, the concept of sound pressure is taken to be variations above or below atmospheric pressure.

Since sound is propagated in (at least) three dimensions, it is important to consider quantities as they apply to masses in three dimensions. Volume is the three-dimensional quantity of a mass, and it is derived by multiplying length by width by depth. The simplest three-dimensional mass is, thus, a cube, whose length, width, and depth are equal, and whose volume (V) is $m \times m \times m$, or m^3.

Three-dimensional masses can be made of any material, including lead, peanut butter, water, or just air. If these materials are formed with the same dimensions, they also have the same volumes. Volume is calculated as the three-dimensional measurement of a mass. In its simplest form, it is expressed as a cube, and measures as the product of the lengths of its three sides, namely, $m \times m \times m$, or m^3. The volume of a sphere is a little more complicated to calculate than the volume of a cube, but is probably more applicable to the propagation of sound in air. The formula for the volume of a sphere is $V = 4/3 \prod r^3$.

It should be clear to all, however, that cubes made of peanut butter do not have the same masses when compared to cubes made of air. They differ in density, or the nature and bonds of molecules of which they are composed and how tightly these molecules are packed next to one another. Density is mass (kg) divided by volume (m^3), and in SI, it is measured in kg/m^3. Volumes made up of differing materials have different densities, and behave accordingly. This includes the way they respond to sound energy.

WORK AND POWER

It takes work to move masses around, even the tiny ones, and the farther they have to be moved, the more work is needed. Just think of the work it takes to move a piano across the room, and then consider moving that same piano around the block. Thus, the physical unit of work is derived as force (N) multiplied by distance or length. This is work in two dimensions. The SI unit

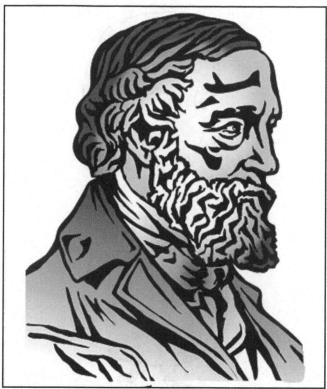

Figure 2-7. James Prescott Joule (1818–1889), for whom the SI unit of work, force × distance, was named, was an English physicist. His studies on the relationship between energy and work might well have been stimulated by practical applications in his family's brewery and led to the principle of conservation of energy or the first law of thermodynamics. The SI unit of pressure is the joule (J). (drawhunter/Shutterstock.com)

of measurement for work is the Nm, or Newton-meter, but work is such an important derived quantity that it has its own unit, the joule, named in honor of British physicist James Prescott Joule (see Figure 2-7). One joule is the amount of work it takes to move a mass of one kilogram over a distance of one meter.

In a similar way, work can be done in three dimensions. It takes work to change the pressure of a gas, such as air, just as it takes work to inflate a balloon. The reverse is true, too: changing the pressure of a gas can create work. Pressure changes in air are examples of work in three dimensions. Similarly, rapid changes in air pressure occur when sound is created. Pressure (N/m^2) multiplied by volume (m^3) is work in three dimensions, and the observant student will note that the derivation still works out to the joule base unit, Newton-meter.

Power is a quantity that describes the time interval over which work is done. It takes more power to do the same amount of work over a longer time, and to do more work over a given time, a more powerful engine is needed. Thus, power is work divided by time, derived as joule/second. The SI unit of power is the watt, named

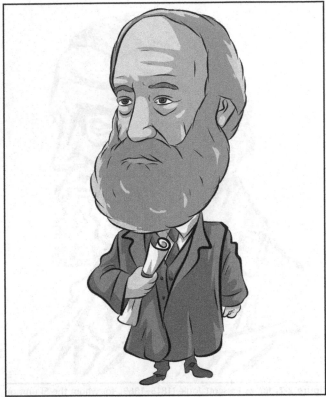

Figure 2-8. James Watt (1736–1819) was a Scottish engineer who invented significant improvements to the steam engine, making it more efficient. The SI unit of power is the watt (W). (molcay/Shutterstock.com)

fundamental and derived quantities used to explain phenomena associated mechanics. It is time to apply these concepts to speech and hearing science. One branch of mechanics is of particular importance for speech, language, and hearing sciences: *acoustics*. Acoustics is the study of sound.

REFERENCES

Clausius, R. (1865). Ueber verschiedene fur die anwendung bequeme formen der hauptgleichungen der mechanischen warmetheorie. *Annalen der Physik, 125,* 353-400. In Wolf, S.L. (2013). Rudolph Clausius-a pioneer of the modern theory of heat. *Vacuum, 90,* 102-108. doi:10.1016/j.vacuum.2012.02.029

Fowler, R. & Guggenheim, E. A. (1939/1965). *Statistical Thermodynamics: a version of statistical mechanics for students of physics and chemistry,* first printing 1939, reprinted with corrections 1965, Cambridge UK: Cambridge University Press.

Kinetic Theory of Gases. (2015). In *Encyclopædia Britannica.* Retrieved from http://www.britannica.com/science/kinetic-theory-of-gases

Mikhailov, G. K. (2005). Daniel Bernoulli, *Hydrodynamica* 1738. In Gratton-Guiness, I. (2005). *Landmark writings in western mathematics 1640-1940* Chapter 9. New York: Elsevier.

National Institute of Standards and Technology (1974). A brief history of measurement systems. *NBS Special Publication 304A.* Retrieved from https://archive.org/stream/briefhistoryuseo304nati#page/n5/mode/2up

Taylor, B. N. & Mohr, P. J. (2015). The NIST reference on constants, units and uncertainty, fundamental physical constants: standard atmosphere. Retrieved from http://physics.nist.gov/cuu/Reference/contents.html

Taylor, B. N. & Thompson, A. (2008). The International system of Units (SI). *NIST Special Publication 330,* 2008 Edition.

for Scottish inventor James Watt (see Figure 2-8). One watt is one joule/second.

We have examined the basics of physics, especially that branch called mechanics, and we have studied

3

Basic Acoustics

GOAL

Familiarize the student with elemental acoustic phenomena for application to speech and language sciences.

OBJECTIVES

- Define sound.
- Distinguish periodic vibration from aperiodic vibration.
- Apply principles of vibration to the concept of waves.
- Distinguish among frequency, period, and amplitude.
- Distinguish pitch from loudness.
- Distinguish sound pressure from intensity.
- Know the minimal sound power level and intensity reference levels for 1,000 Hz.
- Answer questions related to the basic concept underlying the decibel.
- Relate sound pressure to distance of spherical wave propagation.
- Answer questions relating to the basic concept of signal-to-noise ratio.
- Distinguish among time, intensity, periodicity spectrum, and transitions on a speech spectrograph.

• • • • • • •

Culbertson, W. R.
Fundamentals of the Speech and Language Sciences (pp 17-35).
© 2020 Taylor & Francis Group.

SOUND

Sound can be defined as, "A mechanical disturbance from a state of equilibrium that propagates through an elastic material medium" (Encyclopedia Britannica, 2015). From this definition, we can infer that for sound to exist, there must be a material medium through which it can be propagated. The medium can be composed of any material, but air and water are probably the most familiar media to most of us. Media such as air or water are composed of particles called molecules, created by the bonding of atoms. Most of the molecules in air are nitrogen and oxygen, while other gases and water vapor make up the rest of the mixture. An outside energy source is also required to disturb the equilibrium state of molecules in the medium.

A source can be, among many other things, a clap of thunder, a train whistle, a cycling glottis, or a random air disturbance produced by unequal pressure between the loose articulation of the tongue and alveolar ridge. In the case of thunder, the source is a quick expansion of air caused by the heat of lightning. In the case of a train whistle, the source is steam oscillation as it is forced through an aperture especially designed for the purpose. For the glottal sound, the source is pulsing cycles of air pressure variations, and for the alveolar fricative, the source is random disturbance of particle velocity. Whatever the nature of the source, it must be vibrating in a manner within the range of human hearing to produce sounds human beings can hear.

Before the source is applied to the elastic medium, the medium is said to be in a state of equilibrium. In the equilibrium state, molecules that make up the medium are vibrating with respect to one another, just as do all molecules composing masses. However, even though the medium is vibrating, its vibration has reached a steady state and is only changing in the sense that it is approaching entropy. This state of equilibrium can be measured as the atmospheric or barometric pressure. The medium may even be generating sound all by itself, but, at equilibrium, the sound energy is so low that it is hardly noticed.

When the source is applied, it adds its energy to the already vibrating molecules and makes audible sound by disrupting the steady equilibrium state of the material composing the elastic medium. The medium's molecules now vibrate in synchrony with the energy of the source. The natural vibrating characteristics of the particles comprising the medium propagate the disturbance created by the source away from the source's location over distances, the extent of which are determined by the power and other characteristics of the source and the specific elasticity, density, and, to a lesser extent, temperature of the material of the medium.

Source characteristics include the amount of force exerted, with greater force usually associated with greater particle displacement and greater distance of propagation through the medium. Other source characteristics are related to the timing of the source's vibration and the degree to which the source is in natural synchrony with the equilibrium vibrations of the medium.

Elasticity is the degree to which the material resists being deformed. For example, it is a lot easier to deform peanut butter than steel because the strength of the atomic forces holding steel molecules together is greater than those holding peanut butter together. Steel has greater elasticity, and it transmits sound energy much more efficiently than peanut butter. The more elasticity in the material, the greater the degree to which it can respond to the vibrating source, and the faster the speed of sound passing through.

The number of molecules held together in any given mass determines the density of the mass. Ironically, the closer, or denser, the molecules are packed together in a mass, the greater its resistance to the transmission of sound energy, and the slower the speed of sound passing through.

Sound energy is said to *propagate* from its source to other locations, depending upon highly variable conditions. In this sense, propagation means that the source energy that created the disturbance from the equilibrium state moves from one location in the medium to another. Since all the molecules composing the medium are connected by atomic forces, changes in the vibration of one molecule in the medium cause changes in the vibrations of surrounding molecules. These changes affect all the molecules around them, and so on. That means compressions and rarefactions of molecular forces in the medium form layers surrounding the source. These layers of energized molecules push (compress) and pull (rarefy) adjacent molecules in directions away from the sound source location, very much like waves on the ocean. One layer of fully compressed molecules gradually gives way to a layer of completely rarefied molecules. The waves move away from the source location as long as the source continues to vibrate. As one might imagine, the rate and distance of sound propagation vary according to the elastic nature of the medium and the characteristics of the source. When the source stops vibrating, the molecules return to their steady state.

In nature, the direction and other characteristics of sound propagation are not evenly distributed around the source. Many factors may influence them. These factors are the same factors that may influence the density of the medium, such as temperature and the molecular composition of the medium itself. Some media may be so dense that they reflect the energy of propagation. This is particularly true when the energy is propagated from a less dense medium, such as air, to a denser medium, such as cochlear endolymph.

THE SPEED OF SOUND

The rate at which sound propagates through a medium is the speed of sound: distance divided by time, with no directional vector. As one might imagine, this means that the elasticity and density of the medium are crucial to the speed at which sound is propagated. Air and water, both of which are different in density, are the most commonly encountered media through which sound is propagated, at least, external to the skull. Inside the skull, sound is propagated through bone and cochlear fluids, all of which have differing densities to that of air. The relationship between the speed of sound and the elasticity and density of the medium is expressed as the square root of the quotient of elasticity divided by density.

Speed of Sound = $\sqrt{(\text{Elasticity} \div \text{Density})}$

Elastic forces are created by the bonds between molecules composing the medium. These contribute to how much a medium can be deformed by pressure and to how quickly the material returns to its original shape or volume. Thus, the greater the medium's elastic forces, or tightness of its intermolecular bonds, the faster it will propagate sound. Conversely, increasing the material's density will slow the speed of sound. Density, as we have seen, is the amount of material (mass), or the number of molecules, contained within a volume; in other words, density is how closely the molecules are packed together. Temperature is also a factor that must be considered when considering the speed of sound, because heat not only reduces a medium's density, but it also makes the molecules vibrate faster in their equilibrium state. Fast-vibrating molecules transmit sound more quickly than do slow-vibrating molecules.

In dry air, the speed of sound at 20°C is approximately 343 m/sec. In water, at the same temperature, the speed is 1482 m/sec (physicsclassroom.com).

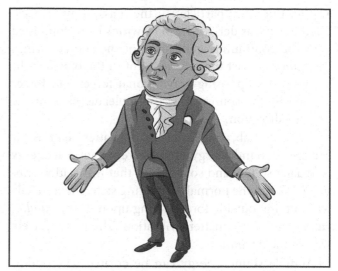

Figure 3-1. Daniel Bernoulli (1700–1782). (molcay/Shutterstock.com)

Sound travels faster in water because the elastic forces in water are stronger than those in air. Note that for both air and water volumes, speed of sound approximations assumes consistent temperature and material composition throughout the medium, a condition almost never observed under natural circumstances. In the natural world, temperature and elevation (depth) variations cause constant changes in the way air and water media conduct sound energy.

The speed and other characteristics of sound depend on the frame of reference. In most cases, we'll call the listener the frame of reference, and we will assume the listener is stationary relative to the sound source. Imagine that a listener is moving away from the source of sound at the same speed as the propagation. In that case, the listener would not hear the sound generated by the source because the sound could not catch up.

SOUND AND VIBRATIONS

The kinetic theory of gases, posited in 1738 by Daniel Bernoulli (Mikhailov, 2005) (see Figure 3-1), stipulates that all the molecular particles in a gas such as air are in constant motion. In fact, particles that comprise all matter vibrate, and the vibration of matter varies according to whether the state of the matter is gaseous, liquid, or solid.

It might simplify matters to imagine these particles, the very molecules that make up the air around us, are moving back and forth about a central point. Whenever a particle moves too far past the central point, gravitational forces generated by the masses of that particle and all the other particles in the mass, draw it back. Then inertia, as derived from Newton's laws, combined with the continuing application of the source, brings the molecule past the central point in the opposite direction until opposing gravitational forces and forces applied by the source draw the molecule back in the original direction.

Normally vibrating particles in matter such as air can create sound energy, but the strength of that energy is usually so low and so constant that it is seldom noticed. We call the normally vibrating state, theoretically without any outside forces acting upon it, the *equilibrium state* of the matter's vibration. The matter, itself, we call the *medium*.

Audible sound energy can be created when additional force of sufficient characteristics is applied from an outside source to the particles at equilibrium in the medium, usually a volume of air. In the case of sound, we are considering additional energy delivered by an outside source to particles already in motion, since particles in all materials vibrate naturally. The application of the outside source energy causes the particles that are already in motion to change their vibratory patterns to correspond with those of the driving source. The energy that causes changes in the normal vibrations of media particles is called *sound energy*, and it is often described as being propagated through vibrations or oscillations of particles in the medium. The term propagation is used because the energy is transferred from one particle to adjacent particles. Although the particles in the medium move back and forth under their own energy and the energy of the outside force, they don't travel very far. Instead, the change in particle vibrations, created by energy, or pressure applied to the volume of air, is transferred from particle to particle within the substance of the medium. This energy is called *acoustic energy*, and acoustic energy generates *sound pressure*.

Application of sound pressure in air compresses and rarefies the particles in the medium, resulting in increases and decreases in the particle density corresponding with increases and decreases in pressure emanating from the source. The additional force of sound pressure may change the rate and/or strength of the normal vibration, and the energy that causes these changes is propagated over distance to include the air molecules in the ear canal of a listener. If the change in vibration is of the proper strength and rate to be within the range of human hearing, the listener will perceive sound.

When the outside force is no longer present, assuming that no more energy is applied, particles will tend to move about in the outside force's vibration patterns until they gradually return to their equilibrium state. The listener will hear no more sound. Imagine the pendulum of a grandfather clock, or the coils of a slinky toy. When you set them in motion, they will move back and forth until you cease to apply outside force, at which point they slow down and stop.

DESCRIPTIVE VIBRATION TERMS

Energy of all kinds is propagated through the known universe in the form of changing particle characteristics. These changes can be thought of as *vibrations*. Particle vibrations can be quite complex, but all forms of vibrations have discernable and measurable characteristics. Vibration characteristics are described in terms of the direction of the vibration relative to the direction of the force applied by the vibrating source, the timing of the changes, the amount of change that occurs, and the array of vibrating characteristics that comprise the source. Vibrations that occur as sound are described by the direction, timing, amount, and array of particle motion in the medium.

Vibratory directions may be one of two types: longitudinal and transverse (see Figure 3-2). Longitudinal vibrations propagate in directions parallel to the direction of the force applied by the source. Sound waves in air propagate with longitudinal vibration, in directions away from the push of the sources. Transverse vibrations occur perpendicular to the direction of the force applied by the source. A vibrating guitar string is a good example of a transverse wave, where the direction of the vibration is along the length of the string, while the plucking motion is usually perpendicular to the length of the string. Light energy also propagates in transverse waves.

Timing parameters of vibrations include *period* and *frequency*. Period is the amount of time it takes the body to complete a single cycle, and frequency is the number of cycles that take place in a given period, usually one second. Since the second is the International System of Units (SI) standard unit of time, it follows that period is quantified in fractions of a second, and frequency is quantified in terms of how many cycles occur in a second. Note that the two time-related parameters are reciprocal: period is seconds/cycle, and frequency is cycles/second. Both period and frequency of sound vibrations are perceived as *pitch*, a psychological

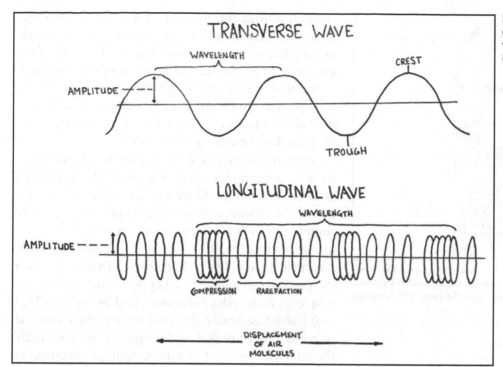

Figure 3-2. Transverse wave propagation compared to longitudinal wave propagation. (Image drawn by Mathew DeVore)

phenomenon that defies quantification but that most listeners can describe as higher or lower relative to a given reference signal.

The amount of particle displacement depends upon how much energy is applied to the medium. In the case of sound, this is perceived as *loudness*. In air, the amount of displacement that occurs is almost always a function of how much pressure is applied by the vibrating source. Sound amplitude is usually measured in *decibels* (dB), a quantity that reflects an observed pressure in comparison with a reference pressure. Loudness is like pitch in being a psychological entity; it's difficult to measure, but noticeable, for most people, in comparison to a reference signal.

While it is convenient to begin the study of sound vibrations in simple terms, as being of a single frequency and of a single amplitude, most wave energy observed in nature is propagated in complex systems. Complex systems have simultaneously occurring multiple components of varying frequencies and amplitudes, and are rarely stable over time. In fact, sound energy propagated at a single frequency, also called a *pure tone*, is rarely (if ever) observed in nature. High quality electroacoustic instruments may get close, but as soon as sound energy is propagated into the atmosphere, harmonic vibration accompanies it, and this creates a complex vibration. In complex systems, vibrations occur at more than one frequency. In some complex systems, the approximate frequencies of an array of multiple component vibrations

can be identified and quantified. In others, only a range of vibrations is identifiable. Either way, the component vibrations make up the *spectrum* of a complex system. Sound spectrum is perceived by listeners as timbre or quality. As an example of the perceptual phenomenon of quality, consider the difference between the same note played on a saxophone and then at the same loudness on a clarinet.

Frequency or period, amplitude and spectrum can vary independently from one another. This means that one can manipulate the frequency of a sound and not change its amplitude or spectrum, or manipulate its amplitude and not change its frequency or spectrum. For example, one can play the middle C note on a clarinet, and then play the same C an octave higher, and not change how loud one plays it. One can also play middle C louder or softer to change its acoustic energy amplitude at the same frequency, or one can play middle C on a saxophone at the same amplitude to change only the spectrum of the complex sound.

TIMING PATTERNS OF VIBRATIONS

Because the pressure of sound is applied to volumes of air over time, the timing of sound energy is of fundamental importance to those who study acoustics. Variations in sound energy wave timing are perceived by listeners as variations in pitch. Pitch is difficult to

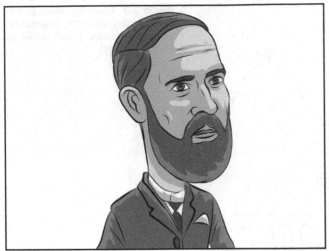

Figure 3-3. Heinrich Hertz (1857–1894) was a German physicist credited with proving that electromagnetic waves, earlier posited by James Maxwell, exist. The standard unit for frequency, the Hertz (Hz), is named after him. (molcay/Shutterstock.com)

measure except in reference to another sound. Timing of vibrations leads us to recognize two types of vibratory timing patterns: *periodic vibration* and *aperiodic vibration*.

PERIODIC VIBRATION

Particles in periodic vibration maintain the same pattern of vibration over successive cycles as long as the same amount of force is exerted upon them. As a theoretical phenomenon, the pattern or pathway of periodic particle vibration can be easily predicted, and this characteristic makes periodic vibration a perfect pattern to begin study.

The trouble is, perfectly periodic vibration has not been observed in the natural world. There are bodies that vibrate very close to exact periodicity, but still not with perfect repetition of cycles. It is, instead, a theoretical concept that is quite useful for study, but not real. Real-world vibration that is almost periodic is properly called *quasi-periodic*, but conventional terminology does away with that distinction and uses the term *pure tone* to designate nearly perfect simple periodic acoustic vibration.

CYCLE

When a vibrating body moves from any position and returns to the same position from the opposite direction, it is said to have completed one cycle of vibration. A particle moving through a vibratory cycle takes a certain amount of time to complete the cycle, just as

anybody moving through space takes time to complete a journey. Remember, the time it takes for a particle to complete one cycle of vibration is the period of the vibration. In SI, the second is the standard time unit, so the time it takes for a particle to complete a cycle is measured in seconds. Thus, if it takes one tenth of a second for a particle to complete one vibratory cycle, the period of the cycle is 0.1 seconds.

Another way to look at the timing of a vibratory cycle is by counting the number of cycles that occur in a given amount of time. Once again, the standard unit for time is the second, and the number of times a particle completes its vibratory cycles in one second is its *frequency* of vibration. If it takes one-tenth of a second for a particle to complete a single cycle of vibration, then the particle can complete 10 cycles in one second. Its frequency is 10 cycles per second, and its period is 1/10 or 0.1 seconds. Notice that frequency is the reciprocal of period. Since period and frequency are essentially the same parameter of vibration, both are perceived as pitch. In honor of Heinrich Hertz, the German physicist (see Figure 3-3), the conventional unit used to specify frequency is the *Hertz*, abbreviated Hz.

PERIOD AND FREQUENCY: TIMING OF VIBRATION

The period of the vibration is the amount of time it takes fluctuations of energy to complete a single cycle, from full compression to full rarefaction and back again, beginning at any point on the scale. Time is represented on the Cartesian projection by the X (horizontal) axis, and is measured in seconds, the SI unit of time. Sound vibrations are so fast, the period is always fractions of a second, or milliseconds.

For example, if a single vibration occurs 1,000 times per second, its period is 0.001 seconds. The frequency of the motion is the number of times the cycle repeats itself per unit of time (usually a full second), and, as mentioned before, is measured in Hz. Higher frequency is depicted by a faster rate of rotation and a shorter period. A listener perceives the frequency or period of a (quasi-) periodic sound as pitch.

Period and frequency are quantities that specify the timing of vibration, and the reader will recall that the International System specified the standard unit for time is the second. The International System uses the nearly perfect vibratory timing of a cesium atom. It specifies the second as the duration of 9,192,631,770 periods of the transition between two hyperfine levels of the ground state of the cesium 133 atom at zero Kelvin (Taylor & Thompson, 2008).

When sound sources vibrate with timing that is nearly periodic, a listener perceives a tone, a musical note, or even the normal human voice producing vowels. Human beings are commonly said to be sensitive to a range of sound frequencies from approximately 20 to 20,000 cycles per second, although because the human ear is most sensitive to sound having frequency between 200 Hz and 8,000 Hz, it takes more energy to make a sound audible at either end of that range. Sound having frequencies below 20 Hz is called *infrasound*, while sound having frequencies above 20,000 Hz is called *ultrasound*.

In a review of the literature on the subject, Moller and Pedersen (2004) reported reliable human responses to sound having frequencies below 20 Hz, but subjects reported that stimuli lost the characteristic of being continuous tones and became more like repetitive tactile sensations. Using electronic acoustic equipment specially designed for the research, Henry and Fast (1984) obtained reliable responses from test subjects to stimuli at frequencies ranging to 24,000 Hz. Audiologists generally use electronically generated, (nearly) pure tones to pinpoint hearing sensitivity across a segment of the range of human hearing from 125 to 8,000 cycles per second (Bess & Humes, 2003).

Both quasi-periodic and aperiodic vibrations are present in speech, produced in various combinations depending upon the speaker. Vowels, approximants, and nasals are produced with variations on the spectra of quasi-periodic complex vibrations, and unvoiced obstruent consonants, including the fricatives and plosives, are variations on aperiodic source spectra. Voiced obstruent consonants are distinguished as mixtures of quasi-periodic and aperiodic spectra.

TYPE OF PHONEME	TYPE OF VIBRATION
Vowels	Quasiperiodic
Approximants	Quasiperiodic
Nasals	Quasiperiodic
Fricatives	
• Unvoiced	• Aperiodic
• Voiced	• Aperiodic plus quasiperiodic
Posives	
• Unvoiced	• Aperiodic
• Voiced	• Aperiodic plus quasiperiodic

AMPLITUDE, PRESSURE, AND INTENSITY: A FUNCTION OF MAGNITUDE

At any given point on its vibratory trip, the vibrating particle is displaced or elongated to some extent. This means that at each instant of time during the cycle, there is a corresponding amount of displacement. The amount of displacement or elongation is a very important parameter of the vibratory pattern, and is called the *amplitude* of the vibration. In air, sound amplitude is a function of the amount of force exerted on a volume of air and is usually quantified as fluctuations in *sound pressure*.

The fact that energy is propagated among particles means that energy fluctuations also occur over time and through areas of the medium. The magnitudes of these energy fluctuations can be measured as *intensity*, or time-averaged energy flux. Intensity amplitudes can be measured in electric circuits as well as in air or any other medium, and the conventional unit is watts per square meter (W/m^2).

Sound pressure and sound intensity, then, are directly related. Greater amplitudes of particle displacement are caused by greater air pressure variations, which are, in turn, caused by greater power (watt) fluctuations over a given area (m^2). Audiological stimuli are most commonly delivered through electronic devices. While intensity can be measured in an electric circuit, sound pressure cannot. However, the intensity of a signal generated through an electronic circuit can be transformed into acoustic energy by reacting with a speaker or earphone. When this happens, the energy becomes transduced into sound pressure. Thus, in electro-acoustic devices, intensity and sound pressure increase and decrease together. Once the acoustic energy stimulates the auditory system, a listener perceives amplitude as loudness.

In studying vibratory patterns of energy forms, including acoustic energy, we can quantify the relative amplitude of particle vibration at any instant during its cycle. In fact, we can examine any characteristic of particle movement, including its distance, amplitude, and acceleration, but the most common parameter measures the amount of particle displacement and its pattern over time.

Amplitude of acoustic energy is related to the personal sensation of loudness. Amplitude means "how

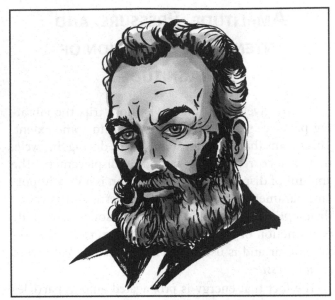

Figure 3-4. Alexander Graham Bell (1847–1922) was an inventor, educator, and scientist who is credited with the original patent for the telephone. Bell is also notable for his work with the deaf and hard-of-hearing community. The Alexander Graham Bell Association for the Deaf and Hard of Hearing is devoted to advancing listening and spoken language for individuals who are deaf and hard of hearing. (Marusya Chaika/Shutterstock.com)

much," and is usually expressed as sound pressure level (SPL) or intensity.

SOUND PRESSURE LEVEL

As you will recall from the lecture on basic physics, pressure is force divided over surface. In acoustics, amplitude is a relative quantity, and is expressed as being above or below ambient conditions. In the case of sound pressure, it is measured above or below ambient or atmospheric pressures.

The SI unit for pressure is the pascal (Pa), equal to a force of one newton applied to a surface of one square meter. Since magnitudes of sound pressure related to human hearing are very small, many hearing scientists cling to the old CGS system by which measurement is in dynes per square centimeter (dynes/cm²) or microbars. Normal atmospheric pressure is 101,325 Pa. This pressure, expressed in dynes, is 1,013,250, or just over one million dynes/cm². Thus, an audible SPL will be that pressure varying over and under approximately 100,000 Pa or 1 million dynes per square centimeter under the normal conditions.

INTENSITY

Intensity is time-averaged energy flux: energy per unit volume divided by the velocity of the energy. A derived quantity, intensity is measured by dividing power (watts) by area (m²). Intensity is not really the same as amplitude, but it is used that way colloquially.

As we have seen, there is a quantifiable relationship between sound pressure and sound intensity. Specifically, the intensity, I, of a sound is proportional to the square of its pressure, p or $I = p^2$. This means that when sound pressure is doubled, intensity does not double. Rather, it is multiplied by a factor of 0.8.

DECIBELS

Sound pressure and intensity are measured in dBs, meaning 10 bels. The bel was named after Alexander Graham Bell (see Figure 3-4), who invented the scale to enable him to work over a wide range of intensities audible to the human ear. Although the word representing his last name is not capitalized and one of the letter "l"s is dropped, interestingly, the first letter of his last name is again capitalized when the word is abbreviated: dB.

To properly study sound amplitudes, Bell needed a measurement scale that would work for the very wide range of sound pressure levels audible to the human ear. Instead of single units like the Pa, Bell devised a scale of natural logarithmic ratios, or expressed as powers of 10, which relate an observed amplitude of sound pressure level or intensity to some arbitrary reference level. Even using the logarithmic scale, a single bel unit was not enough, so Bell worked in 10-bel units that ultimately became dBs. The dB scale was a success, and it is used to this day. It expresses sound amplitude as a ratio, one SPL or intensity over a reference level, rather than a standard unit. The two amplitude levels compared are, however, expressed in standard units, such as Pa or watts.

Since the scale is a ratio, the dB formula is $10 \log_{10}$ of the value to be compared divided by the value of the reference level. The 10 multiplier reflects the need to work in dBs rather than bels, and the 10 subscript indicates the logarithmic base 10, working in powers of 10, of the natural logarithm.

REFERENCE LEVELS FOR DECIBELS

Alert readers will note that a dB means nothing unless the reference level is specified. Unless a reference level is understood or previously established in writing, or even in conversation, the reference level is always expressed right after the term dB is used.

The American National Standards Institute established standard reference levels for sound intensity of a just audible 1,000 Hz tone in the early 1930s. Fletcher and Munson (1933) related the then-proposed standard intensity reference level of 10^{-16} watts/cm^2 (1^{-11} watts/m^2) to a sound pressure level of 0.000207 dynes/cm^2, now quantified in SI as 10^{-5} Pa. The reference level for intensity is 1^{-11} watts/m^2, or 10^{-16} watts/cm^2 in older literature. These reference levels are still in conventional use today.

Thus, when specifying a reference level of 2×10^{-5} Pa for sound pressure, it is appropriate to add the phrase, "re: 2×10^{-5} Pa/square meter, or simply SPL, after the quantity."

NOISE AND SIGNAL

Noise may be described as any sound that interferes with the detectability of another. In speech acoustics, we are concerned that noise, present in almost any environment, doesn't make our speech signal unintelligible.

Signal-to-noise ratio is the relationship of the amplitudes of a signal of interest to a background noise. Obviously, the ratio of signal-to-noise is best if our signal of interest is sufficiently large enough that our listener can ignore the noise and tune in to the signal.

Since dBs are ratios and signal-to-noise is a ratio, we can express signal-to-noise ratio as a number of dBs. The higher the number of dBs, the easier it will be to listen to the signal and ignore the noise.

DAMPENED VIBRATION

As long as the same force is applied to an object in vibration, it will continue to vibrate in a constant pattern. In reality, force varies in amplitude over time. If the force originally applied to a body in vibration subsides, then the extent of that body's pattern of excursion will lessen with time, and if that force increases, so will the extent of excursion. Remember the grandfather clock? Without the force applied to the clockworks by the hanging weights, the pendulum gradually stops swinging. This may occur because of changes in the source or changes in the medium.

Dampened, also called damped, vibration is simply vibration that fades away, or decreases in strength. It is not necessary that the movement patterns remain constant. In fact, acoustic energy in the natural world rarely does, and most vibratory patterns fade away at a relatively quick rate.

SIMPLE HARMONIC MOTION

The most basic type of vibration is *simple harmonic motion* (SHM). The term SHM describes a single periodic vibratory pattern over time, having a single period and frequency and a single maximum amplitude. Acoustically, SHM would be perceived as a pure tone, or as close as possible to a pure tone as the listener's auditory system would permit.

That means that, just like a pure tone or a perfect periodic vibration, SHM is a laboratory concept, nearly impossible to find beyond the scientific imagination. Modern electronic instrumentation can get close, but is still not perfect, especially once a sound is transduced from electronic energy to acoustic energy with a speaker. However, the concept of SHM is of great value as a foundation for the study of more complex vibratory patterns.

Accordingly, we will consider SHM to occur only along a straight line and in only two dimensions. That should make it clear how abstract our ideal SHM concept is. The particle travels from the original resting or equilibrium position, which we will call zero, to the point of maximum displacement, which we will designate as A+, then back through zero to a negative displacement equal to the positive displacement, A-, and back to zero to complete one cycle.

GRAPHING SIMPLE HARMONIC MOTION

A key concept in studying SHM is to compare its recurrent fluctuations to points on a circle. Like a rider on a merry-go-round, the values of energy fluctuation wax and wane, taking on the same values with each journey around the circle. Sometimes the journey is called uniform circular motion. It is easy to see how each complete repetition of energy fluctuations can be called a *cycle*. The time it takes to complete a turn is called the period.

An excellent means of studying SHM is by examining a Cartesian graph of the cyclic changes in energy over time. The graph is simply the projection of points on the circumference touched by a rotating ray to a Cartesian coordinate graph (see Figure 3-5). Such a graph can depict any variation in the perfectly cycling energy, but most often the graph represents cyclic amplitude variations. In its most commonly seen form, the horizontal X-axis, or abscissa, shows time, and the vertical Y-axis, or ordinate, shows the amplitude of particle displacement at any instant around the circle. Time is the independent variable, meaning we can change its

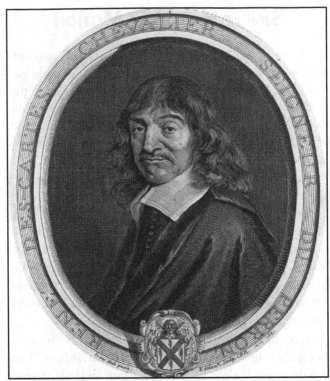

Figure 3-5. René Descartes (1596–1650) invented the Cartesian coordinate graphic system.

value at any instant to be whatever we want, and the amount of particle displacement is dependent upon whatever time we choose. Since the acoustic energy we are studying now varies over time in a perfectly continuous and exactly repetitive compression and rarefaction pattern, we can describe the energy variations in terms of a perfect circle, and project the variations to a linear graph.

The result will be a uniformly wavy *sinusoidal curve* showing the relative displacement of a given particle at any instant over the period of the cycle. The curve varies above and below the abscissa as the uniform circular motion designates regular compressions and rarefactions of the cyclic energy source.

The curve is called sinusoidal because it is identical to the graphic curve that is created when we plot the trigonometric sine (pronounced, /saIn/) function of an angle, changing as the amplitude of particle displacement changes, in uniform circular patterns, or cycles, over time. In trigonometry, the sine function describes the ratio of the lengths of lines created by extending rays from the center of a circle to its circumference. A *ray* is a line extending from the center of a circle to its circumference, and we can imagine a ray circling around the circle like a stopwatch hand at a constant

rate, completing a round trip in exactly the same amount of time for every cycle.

If we extend a ray from the circle's center to the circle's edge just before the instant the energy starts cycling, and freeze another ray in time at some other instant during the cycle, we will have traced two rays, and there will be an angle between them. Since common notation for a circle allows 360 degrees around the circumference, it is convenient to note the point of the intersection of the first ray with the circle's circumference, just before the cycle starts, as zero degrees.

Now, the graph can be set in motion. We imagine the second rotating ray as moving around the circle at a constant rate, one cycle for every period. Remember, the period is the amount of time it takes to complete a cycle. The second ray will touch the circumference at any real number of degrees around the 360-degree circle, and the angle formed between the two lines is of that number of degrees. The vertex of the angle is the center of the circle. The angle can be large or small, depending on when the cycle is frozen, and the point at which the second ray intersects the circle represents the exact instant in the cycle's period we wish to examine the energy's fluctuation. Extending a perpendicular line from the rotating ray, wherever it is on the circumference, to intersect the ray extended at zero degrees creates a triangle. If we imagine the rotating ray constantly moving, we can also imagine that the length of the perpendicular line will constantly change as well.

Trigonometry is the study of triangles formed by rays extending through circles. The *sine function* is the ratio of the length of the perpendicular line to the length of the second rotating ray, measured from the center of the circle to the edge of the circle. It is easy to see that the length of the perpendicular line will vary constantly as the second ray moves uniformly around the circle, and the point at which it touches the first, or zero, ray will vary constantly over time as well. The same can be said about the ratio of the perpendicular line's length to the length of the rotating line. The length of the rotating ray, however, will remain exactly the same as the length of the zero ray. The angle between the two rays will also vary constantly as the second ray moves around the circle. If we plot the sine function on a Cartesian coordinate graph, using the X-axis to represent the flow of time, and the Y-axis to represent particle displacement or pressure, the result will be the familiar curvy line we call the *sine wave*. The graphic curve of our uniform circular motion is called sinusoidal because it represents the curve of the trigonometric function, sine (see Figure 3-6).

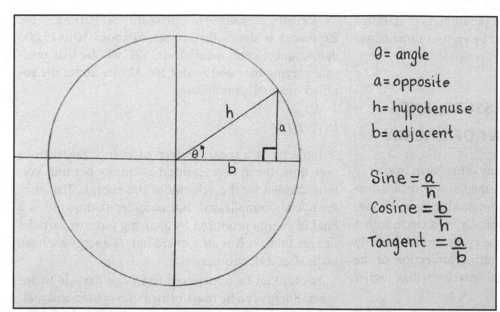

Figure 3-6. A line projected from the center of a circle to any point on its perimeter can be the hypotenuse of a triangle. (Redrawn by Mathew DeVore from http://mathworld.wolfram.com/Sine.html)

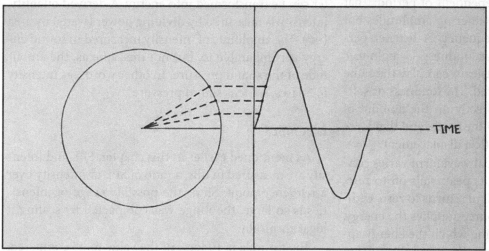

Figure 3-7. Linear projection of radius points on the circumference of a circle forms a sinusoidal wave on a Cartesian graph. Time is the X-axis and amplitude is the Y-axis. (Image drawn by Mathew DeVore)

Setting the cycle in motion, we can extend lines from the rotating ray to create a Cartesian graph that looks just like the graph of a SHM. One line can extend from the vertex of the angle out to the right as far as we wish to measure. This will represent time, our independent variable. We begin at zero, and the farther we go along the line, the longer will be the time we wish to measure. The time line will also represent the position of our vibrating body at equilibrium. The vertical coordinate will represent cyclic fluctuations of whatever dependent variable we intend to examine, dependent upon time. Most of the time, this parameter is the amplitude of pressure variation.

If we draw lines parallel to the time line from the cycling ray out to the right at several instances or phases of the cyclic rotation (see Figure 3-7), we will notice that the lines first rise, then fall back toward the time line, passing through and below the time line, then rising back toward the time line to start another cycle. Dependent variable linear projection points rise then fall, then pass through the time line, only to return and repeat the cycle. The projected line will look like a perfect wave, rising equally above and below the independent variable line, perfectly repeating itself every cycle.

Since we are studying a single example of SHM, the hypotenuse length will remain constant. The length of the line opposite the angle will increase as the ray rotates, decrease to zero, become negative, increase back to zero, and increase again in a uniform cycle. Since sine is a ratio, units are not involved. Further, its value will increase from zero to 1.0 (or -1.0).

Thus, the graph of SHM in acoustics representing a theoretical pure tone is a sine wave. It is important to remember that the sine wave is a graph depicting varying values as functions of time, and not representing the actual movements of particles as they travel through the medium. Several important parameters of uniform circular motion are represented by various dimensions of the graph.

AMPLITUDE, PRESSURE, AND INTENSITY: AMOUNT OF ENERGY

The amplitude of sound or any other form of energy is the amount of energy transformed at any instant during its propagation. A greater amplitude of particle displacement is represented graphically by a circle with a larger radius when we project the cyclic motion linearly as a function of time. The resulting projection of the circular motion in a sinusoidal waveform has higher peaks and deeper valleys.

Note that amplitude is independent of period. That is, we can have waveforms of differing amplitudes but with the same period and frequency. A listener perceives amplitude of vibration as loudness. Using music as an analogy, recall that a musician can play the same pitch as soft or as loud as desired. The loudness or softness of the music depends directly on the amount of force the musician uses to play the notes, and that force determines the amount of particle displacement.

The amplitude of a sinusoidal waveform varies continuously. Amplitude reaches its peak, falls off to zero, descends to the negative peak and returns to zero, without stopping, as long as the source supplies the energy. The portion of the period during which the energy approaches its peak is called its *rise time*, and the portion during which it returns to zero is called its *fall time*. After zero, even though the energy is approaching its maximum negative value, the approach is still called rise time.

Amplitude of acoustic energy is that parameter related to the sensation of loudness. Amplitude is usually expressed as sound pressure level (SPL) or intensity.

SOUND PRESSURE LEVEL

As you will recall from the lecture on basic physics, pressure is force divided over surface. In acoustics, we measure amplitude as a relative quantity, expressed above or below ambient conditions. Thus, sound pressure is measured above and below ambient or atmospheric pressures. The SI unit for pressure is the newton meter-squared (N/m^2) or Pa. For many years, acoustic scientists traditionally used the old CGS system, in which the measurement standard was dynes/cm^2.

Normal atmospheric pressure is 101,325 Pa. Expressed as dynes that comes to about 101,325,000 dynes/square centimeter. Thus, SPL will be that pressure varying over and under 101,325 Pa under the so-called "normal" conditions.

INTENSITY

Intensity is a measurement of energy fluctuations over time. It can be measured as energy per unit volume divided by the velocity of the energy. That may seem a bit complicated, but consider that sound is a kind of energy produced by applying force to particles in a medium such as air. Other kinds of energy are heat, nuclear, and electromagnetic.

Energy can be transferred from one particle to another. Energy can be transformed into matter, and matter can be transformed into energy. A derived quantity, intensity is measured by dividing power (watts) by area (m^2). The amplitude of intensity measured in sound energy is comparable to, but not the same as, the amplitude of the sound pressure. In other words, as intensity increases, so does sound pressure.

DECIBELS

As mentioned earlier in this chapter, SPL and intensity are measured in dBs, a ratio of SPL or intensity over a reference point. Since the possible range of intensities is so large, the range was compacted by scaling it logarithmically.

The formula is $10 \log_{10}$ of the value to be compared, divided by the value of the reference point; in other words, "10 times the natural logarithm of the amplitude to be measured, divided by the natural logarithm of a reference value." If the reference value is 2×10^{-5} Pa, it is expressed as dBspl.

The alert reader will notice right off that the level of dBs reported is pretty meaningless unless the value of the reference is reported. That means that the total number of dBs depends on the value of the reference, and that the reference MUST be reported along with the number of dBs.

REFERENCE LEVELS FOR DECIBELS

The standard reference point for acoustics is the minimum SPL or intensity levels at which a 1,000 Hz tone is barely audible. Fletcher and Munson (1933) chose this level rather arbitrarily based on standards proposed by a subcommittee of the American Standards

Association, now the American National Standards Institute. This level is 10^{-11} watts/m² for intensity, which translates into 2×10^{-5} Pa of sound pressure when sound is delivered through headphones. For many years, intensity and sound pressure references were reported in the old CGS system as 2×10^{-4} dynes/cm² for SPL and 10^{-16} watts/cm² for intensity.

As mentioned above, there is a relation between sound pressure and intensity. Specifically, the intensity of a sound is proportional to the square of its pressure: $I = P^2$. This means that when sound pressure is doubled, intensity does not double. Rather, it is multiplied by a factor of 0.8.

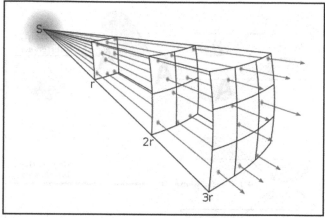

Figure 3-8. Portion of spherical projection of energy from a power source shows surface increase and power decrease. ("Inverse square law.svg" by Borb / used under CC BY-SA 3.0 / Desaturated from original)

INVERSE SQUARE LAW: SOUND AMPLITUDE AND DISTANCE

We all have observed in everyday life that loudness diminishes as a function of distance from the source. It is harder to understand or even hear a speaker as you move farther away. This phenomenon is expressed algebraically as The Law of Inverse Squares. This law stipulates that intensity of energy decreases as the inverse square of distance: $I_2/I_1 = (D_1/D_2)^2$.

This law is understandable when sound is radiating as a spherical pattern (see Figure 3-8). The surface of a sphere is the square of its radius. However, since $I = P^2$, (intensity is equal to the square of pressure) the relationship of sound pressure level to distance is represented as follows: $P_1/P_2 = D_1/D_2$.

At a distance of one meter, conversational speech has a sound pressure of about 60 dBSPL, while a vacuum cleaner generates about 70 dBSPL. See: http://www.sengpielaudio.com/TableOfSoundPressureLevels.htm.

NOISE AND SIGNAL-TO-NOISE RATIO

We have seen in the section on basic acoustics that noise may be described as any sound that interferes with the detectability of another. For that matter, any signal of any form that interferes with the detectability of another signal can be considered noise. In speech acoustics, we are concerned that acoustic noise, present in almost any environment, doesn't make our speech signal unintelligible.

Signal-to-noise ratio is the relationship of the amplitudes of a signal of interest to a background noise. Obviously, the ratio of signal-to-noise is best if our signal of interest is sufficiently large that our listener can ignore the noise and tune in to the signal.

Since dBs are ratios, and signal-to-noise is a ratio, we can express the signal-to-noise ratio as a number of dBs without referring to a reference level. In this case, the noise level is the reference level, and the signal amplitude is directly compared to the noise level. It doesn't really matter what the actual dB reference levels are, such as 10^{-5} Pa/m², for the signal or for the noise, since the real reference in this parameter is the noise.

If we calculate a signal-to-noise ratio of 10 dB, it means that the signal is 10 dB greater in amplitude than the noise. A signal–to-noise ratio can be negative, too, meaning the noise is louder than the signal. If a noise is 10 dB louder than the signal, then the signal-to-noise ratio is -10 dB. If the ratio is zero dB, then both signal and noise are of equal strength. Obviously, the higher the signal-to-noise ratio, the easier it is for a listener to hear and perceive the signal and to ignore the noise.

PHASE

In graphing SHM, *phase* is the number of degrees defining the angle at any instant in the cycle. Up to now, we have considered propagating an SHM at zero degrees, the very instant that the energy begins compressing air particles from their steady state. However, SHMs can begin at any instant of a period, and the beginning instant is described as the number of degrees in the angle defining the place on the cycle. SHM can begin at zero degrees or any other number of degrees up to 360 or zero degrees.

In the real world of sound production, phase becomes most relevant when listeners can perceive it. A

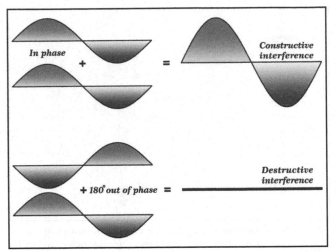

In phase **+** **=** *Constructive interference*

+ 180° out of phase = *Destructive interference*

Figure 3-9. Combinations of SHMs in phase, 90 degrees out of phase, 180 degrees out of phase. (Fouad A. Saad/Shutterstock.com)

single periodic sound can begin at any phase point, and listeners cannot perceive any difference. Listeners can perceive phase when two or more quasiperiodic waves of differing phases are propagated at the same time. When this happens, the resulting energy form is no longer a SHM. Instead, combining two or more SHMs creates a *complex wave*. In such cases, the energy variations affect the amplitude of the combined waveform. Depending upon the amount of difference in their phases, combining SHMs of differing phases can decrease or dampen the resulting sound's amplitude to varying extents, even to the point of cancelling audible sound altogether, or they can combine to the point of doubling the sound's peak amplitude (see Figure 3-9). Combining SHMs of differing phases can also increase the resulting wave to varying extents, even to the point of doubling the resulting sound's amplitude.

Two other familiar circumstances offer listeners opportunities to perceive phase variations. The most usual of these occurs when listeners localize sound origins. One component of this generally automatic central nervous system function is the unconscious detection of slight phase differences that occurs as sound reaches one ear slightly later than it reaches the other. Another common instance in which phase differences affect the average listener is when room acoustics result in sound energy reflection, and waves emanating from a source meet similar waves reflecting from a wall near a 180-degree differential, dampening the acoustic energy enough to cause a dead zone in the room, where listeners have difficulty hearing the source.

COMPLEX WAVES

In reality, not much is pure. This is as true for energy forms as it is with most other phenomena. Thus, the sounds we hear in the world around us, including the sounds of speech, are formed by combinations of multiple sound sources, including some with nearly periodic energy and some with random, aperiodic energy. These sound waves are called complex waves.

The characteristics of the sound energies that combine to form a complex wave comprise the spectrum of the resulting wave. Each individual energy is called a *component* of the spectrum. Listeners perceive spectra as *quality* or *timbre*.

Imagine a single musical note a musician might play on several different instruments, including a trumpet, a clarinet, and a saxophone, with one no louder than the other. For an example, we choose middle C, which has a frequency of 256 Hz. As played on different instruments, these notes have the same basic frequency and amplitude, but they are easily identified as different because of their different spectra. All sound energy with multiple vibrating components will have spectra, whether or not the energy is periodic. In speech, spectra are the distinguishing acoustic features for the categorical discrimination of most phonemes, and they are essential to a listener's understanding of the sounds of speech.

COMBINING SIMPLE HARMONIC MOTIONS

When SHM waves are propagated at the same time, the result is a complex periodic wave. The frequency or period and the amplitude of combined SHMs are easily predicted. The resulting wave form is simply the sum of the parameters of the components at each instant of the cycle. That is, the amplitudes at every instant over each component's cycle can be added and plotted on a Cartesian coordinate graph, in the same way any SHM is plotted. Note that the wave form is still recurring, and is, thus, nearly periodic.

For example, a combination of two SHMs of the same frequency and amplitude, both beginning at the same instant or phase, will be a wave with the same frequency as the original two and having twice the amplitude as each component. This makes sense, since two power sources are working together at the same time.

Their amplitudes at any given time simply add together (see Figure 3-10).

The same principle holds true if the two component waves begin at different phases. If the component waves are equal in frequency and amplitude, but one begins compressing air particles while the other begins by rarefying air particles, they are said to be 180 degrees out-of-phase. For every positive compression of particles one component produces, the other one will produce a corresponding rarefaction of those particles at the same instant. The resulting energy of one component will cancel the energy of the other component, and there will be no sound. By the same principle, if two otherwise identical components are 90 degrees out of phase, the result will be a wave with an amplitude of half of the component waves.

Any number of SHMs of any parameters can combine in the same way (see Figure 3-11). The resulting wave form has multiple components, and the frequency of the combined wave will always be equal to the frequency of the lowest component frequency. The waveform of combinations of more and more SHMs begins to look less and less wavy, and the graph of a theoretical energy source with an infinite number of components is called a *square wave* (see Figure 3-12). A square wave has an instantaneous rise and fall time, with peak energies forming a flat duration along the abscissa. No matter how many components a complex periodic waveform has, however, its frequency will still be the same frequency as the lowest component.

The lowest component of a complex wave is called its *fundamental frequency* or, sometimes, just, *the fundamental*. It is denoted F_0 (physical notation, used by speech and hearing scientists) or f_1 (musical notation). Component energies other than the fundamental are called *harmonics of the fundamental*, or just *harmonics*, and are denoted F_1, F_2, F_3, and so on, to F_n.

Harmonic frequencies are integral, or whole number, multiples of the fundamental frequency, and the fundamental is the largest integral dividend of the harmonics. If the fundamental is 100 Hz, and the components are 300 Hz and 700 Hz, then the components are called the third and seventh harmonics of the fundamental.

Since a complex wave is a combination of its components, the components of a complex wave can be determined by performing a Fourier analysis of the waveform. This is a powerful technique, using complex algorithms, the mechanics of which are beyond the scope of this course. Fourier analysis is named for Jean-Baptiste Joseph Fourier, a French mathematician and engineer (1768 to 1830) (see Figure 3-13).

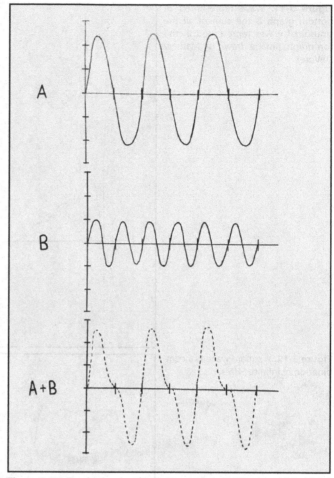

Figure 3-10. Combining amplitude/time graph of A (top) and B (middle) results in graph C (bottom), the sum of A and B. Note that the frequency of C is the same as that of A. (Image drawn by Mathew DeVore)

GRAPHING SPECTRA

A graph is simply a linear representation of a fraction, one value divided by (per) another. Other graphic representations represent other ways of studying sound energy. While the Cartesian waveform graph is useful for representing energy variations over time, a graphic depiction of spectrum is also revealing. Simply put, a spectrum is an array of values measured at any given instant.

For example, a power spectrum graph is often used to represent how much power is generated by each of the various components of a complex wave. This form of spectrum plots amplitude over frequency, showing the relative amplitudes of the component frequencies of a complex wave. The abscissa shows the frequencies, and the ordinate shows the power amplitudes of each component. In a two-dimensional power spectrum, time is not part of the picture.

Figure 3-11. Wave represented in bottom graph is the sum of all the sinusoidal waves represented in the top graph. (Image drawn by Mathew DeVore)

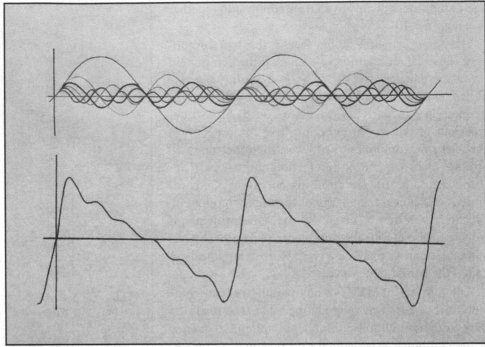

Figure 3-12. A square wave is a combination of infinite SHMs.

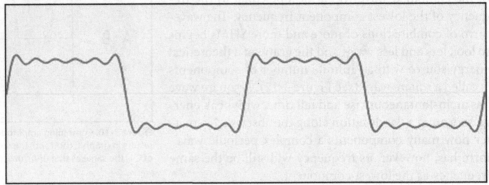

The simplest version of the power spectrum would be that of a pure tone. It would show a single vertical bar, rooted at the specified frequency and rising to the appropriate amplitude shown on the abscissa. Additional components are represented by additional vertical bars, each at its specified frequency and rising to the specified amplitude.

Phase is not represented with a power spectrum. Instead, it is represented with a phase spectrum, with frequency on the abscissa and phase angle, in degrees or radians, represented on the ordinate.

APERIODIC VIBRATION

Aperiodic vibration has no timing parameters other than the period duration between its beginning and its end (see Figure 3-14). There is no single frequency or formant band. Aperiodic vibration instead varies its compressions and rarefactions in a random way, and there is no way to predict its temporal vibratory parameters at any given instant by examining previous energy fluctuations. Examples of aperiodic vibration in the world around us include the hissing sound emanating from a fan, the pop of an exploding balloon, and the unvoiced fricative and plosive sound of speech.

Aperiodic sounds do have spectra, though, just as other complex sounds have. In the case of aperiodic vibration, there is no clear distinction between the component frequencies. Instead, the spectrum of complex, aperiodic sound is said to be *continuous*, with lower frequencies blending smoothly and without interruption into higher frequencies. In contrast to the continuous spectra of aperiodic sound, the spectra of periodic or quasiperiodic sounds are said to be *discrete*, meaning there are clear distinctions between the frequencies of component waves. Since aperiodic sound has no single frequency, acoustic scientists describe the energy in

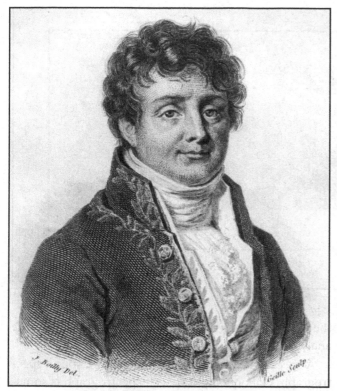

Figure 3-13. Joseph Fourier (1768–1830) proposed the basis for the analysis of complex energy waves, including those of sound, by studying heat energy transfer. This resulted in the principle that any periodic function could be analyzed in terms of an infinite series of component periodic functions, whether or not it was composed of discrete or continuous spectra (Weisstein, 2016). Fourier promoted the French Revolution (1789 to 1799) and was nearly executed during the subsequent Reign of Terror. He was scientific advisor to Napoleon Bonaparte, specializing in Egyptian studies. When Napoleon fell from power, Fourier became a prominent academic figure, appointed to the Académie des Sciences, the Académie Française, and the Académie Nationale de Médecine (Encyclopædia Britannica, 2016).

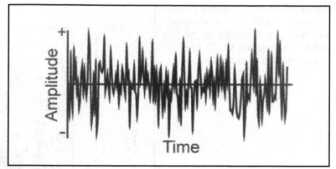

Figure 3-14. Graph of aperiodic wave.

terms of its frequency range, often called its *bandwidth*, with a low end and a high end, and no discrete values within the band.

When sound sources vibrate without periodicity, the listener perceives something commonly called *noise*. Most people think of noise as something we hear, but the term is often used to describe any sensation, auditory or otherwise, that obscures or confuses perception of any signal of interest. In the present context, the noise is auditory. Aperiodic sound with a broad frequency range is called *wide-band noise*, and contrasts with *narrow-band noise*, which has its lowest frequency closer to its highest frequency.

The power spectra of acoustic noise can have different characteristics. Most of the variations are in bandwidth and upon the amplitude characteristics within its energy range. Aperiodic sound having equal energy at all frequencies within human hearing range is called *white* or Gaussian noise. *Pink* noise has energy that decreases (dampens) at a rate of 3 dB (pressure level) per octave, whenever a frequency point is half the value of a previous one. Narrow band noise, used routinely by audiologists to mask the contralateral ear in pure tone threshold testing, has a center frequency equal to that of the pure tone stimulus delivered to the test ear, with a band of gradually attenuated acoustic energy above and below the center frequency.

Two important examples of aperiodic vibration are observed in speech and can be distinguished by their durations. One is described as transient, occurring only over a very brief or instantaneous duration, and the other is described as continuous, sustained over as long a duration as a speaker wishes. Transient aperiodic energy is created during plosive articulation, while continuous aperiodic energy is created during fricative articulation. For example, the transient aperiodic sound propagated during articulation of the plosive phoneme, /p/, when uttered as a syllable releaser, has a power spectrum with most energy ranging from 500 Hz to 1,500 Hz and a duration of around 0.105 seconds. In contrast, the aperiodic continuous sound created during /s/ articulation has most of its energy in a bandwidth from around 3,000 Hz to more than 8,000 Hz, and a typical duration of 0.129 seconds (Edwards, 2003; Crystal & House, 1988; Umeda, 1977).

SPEECH SPECTROGRAPHY

One major problem inhibiting the scientific study of speech is time. Since speech is conveyed by sound, and sound energy quickly fades away from observation, scientists have tried multiple ways of freezing it in time to study it. The problem was how to make fleeting speech "stand still."

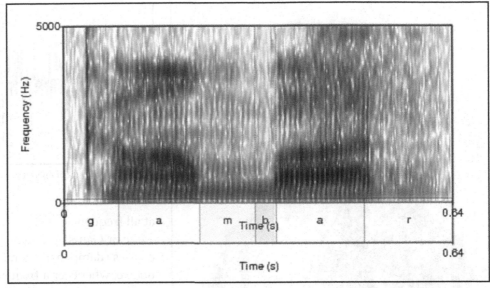

Perhaps the first successful way to make a spoken word linger for serious study was writing in some form. Writing has proven to be an excellent way to preserve the content of speech, but is lacking in its use to preserve the actual sounds of speech for acoustic study. How nice it would be to actually hear the voices of famous figures in history!

Another major milestone in this effort has been phonetic transcription. Transcription captures the segmental and, to some extent, the suprasegmental aspects of the spoken word, but it is heavily dependent upon the skills, the observations, and, unfortunately, the academic predispositions of the transcriber as well as the reader. At that, there is still much left to the imagination.

Audio and video recordings of speakers are another great step in the right direction, but they, too, are transient, even though they can be replayed. However, a developmental offspring of audio recording has extended the usefulness of that modality: *speech spectrography*.

The spectrum of speech is perhaps the most important perceptual characteristic determinant of its purpose: that of conveying meaning as a language modality. As such, speech scientists pay special attention to spectral features of speech acoustics. These features vary constantly over time as the speech articulators are in constant motion over the duration of an utterance.

A *sound spectrograph* produces a visual representation of sound as it occurs over time. In a typical spectrograph, time is represented on the abscissa, and frequency is represented on the ordinate (see Figure 3-15). Amplitude is represented by the darkness of the tracing or, in more recent examples, by the color of the visual display. Probably the most productive use of the sound spectrograph is to provide a vehicle for the analysis of speech.

A speech spectrogram is produced by a sound spectrograph. Colloquially, a speech spectrograph is sometimes called a voiceprint. By either name, it is a visual representation of the acoustics of a spoken signal as it occurred over time, with time represented on the abscissa and frequency represented on the ordinate.

Early speech spectrographs transduced energy stored as magnetic variations on a segment of audio tape, and literally burned these variations onto a piece of special paper. The duration of the speech being analyzed was directly related to the length of the audio tape segment to be analyzed, and was most typically 2.4 seconds. The length of this tape segment corresponded, in turn, to the length of paper upon which it was projected. Amplitude was represented by the darkness of the paper imprint, since voltage passed through a metallic stylus pressed against the special paper varied as a function of signal amplitude, actually burning a darker image on the special paper as the signal amplitude voltage, with subsequent smoke and ash as byproducts. Frequency was represented on the ordinate after the audio recording signal passed through a preprogrammed Fourier analysis device. Frequency could be specified continuously by ordinate values, and two variations of the original spectrograms were the so-called wide-band and narrow-band spectrographs, depending on the range of frequencies represented by the spectrogram. Paradoxically, the wide-band display actually shows a narrower frequency bandwidth than the narrow-band display, with a typical range of about 4,000 Hz, compared to a frequency range of more than

8,000 for the narrow-band display. In this case, the term *wide-band* refers to the fact that formant bands can be shown on a graph with broader physical widths in the more limited frequency range.

Modern spectrograms are produced digitally on screens by more sophisticated computers, without the smoke and ash of yesteryear. The basic parameters of frequency, amplitude, and time are still shown in the same dimensions as they were shown on the originals.

Frequency is still represented as values on the ordinate. In speech, where there is a quasiperiodic source present, such as when vowels, approximants, nasals, or voiced obstruents are uttered, the source is represented as horizontal bands called *formants*. Since the vocal tract has several resonant frequencies, several of these formants will appear, and their relative positions will vary depending upon the shape of the recorded speaker's vocal tract from moment to moment. Formant bands will extend horizontally for a distance equivalent to the time during which the quasiperiodic source was present in the original recording. When an aperiodic source is present, such as when fricatives or plosives are uttered, the spectrograph will show a wide band of sound energy, with no particular distinction between the lower and upper frequency ranges. Voiced fricatives will show a combination of the wide, indistinct aperiodic energy band, combined with identifiable formant bands inside the aperiodic range.

Amplitude is most often represented by colors, with hot colors such as red or orange representing higher amplitudes, and cooler blues and greens showing at the lower amplitude ends of the scales. All these visual representations are positioned according to the times during the recording at which they began and ended.

Since frequency, amplitude, and temporal information are already encoded as part of the digitized acoustic record, observers have only to move on-screen cursors to desired locations on the visual spectrographic image to study parameters recorded at any selected instant, and to tarry there as long as needed.

REFERENCES

Bess, F. H., & Humes, L. E. (2003). Audiology: The fundamentals. Philadelphia, PA: Lippincott, Williams & Wilkins.

Crystal, T. H., & House, A. S. (1988a). The duration of American-English vowels: an overview. *Journal of Phonetics, 16*, 263-284.

Crystal, T. H., & House, A. S. (1988b). The duration of American-English stop consonants: an overview. *Journal of Phonetics, 16*, 285-294.

Edwards, H. T. (2003). *Applied phonetics: The sounds of American English* (3rd ed.). Clifton Park, NY: Delmar Learning.

Fletcher, H., & Munson, G. W. A. (1933). Loudness, its definition, measurement and calculation. *Journal of the Acoustical Society of America, 5*, 82-108.

Henry, K. R., & Fast, G. A. (1984). Ultrahigh-frequency auditory thresholds in young adults: Reliable responses up to 24kHz with a quasi-free-field technique. *Audiology, 23*, 477-489.

Joseph, Baron Fourier. (2016). In *Encyclopædia Britannica*. Retrieved from http://www.britannica.com/biography/Joseph-Baron-Fourier

Kinetic Theory of Gases. (2015). In *Encyclopædia Britannica*. Retrieved from http://www.britannica.com/science/kinetic-theory-of-gases

Mikhailov, G. K. (2005). Daniel Bernoulli, *Hydrodynamica* 1738. In Gratton-Guiness, I. (2005). *Landmark writings in western mathematics 1640-1940*, Chapter 9. New York: Elsevier.

Moller, H., & Pedersen, C. S. (2004). Hearing at low and infrasonic frequencies. *Noise Health, 6*, 37-57. Retrieved from http://www.noise-andhealth.org/text.asp?2004/6/23/37/31664

Sound. (2015). In *Encyclopædia Britannica*. Retrieved from http://www.britannica.com/science/sound-physics

Taylor, B. N., & Mohr, P. J. (2015). The NIST reference on constants, units and uncertainty, fundamental physical constants: standard atmosphere. Retrieved from http://physics.nist.gov/cuu/Reference/contents.html

Taylor, B. N., & Thompson, A. (2008). The international system of units (SI). *NIST Special Publication 330*, 2008 Edition.

the Physics Classroom (1996-2015). The speed of sound. Retrieved from http://www.physicsclassroom.com/class/sound/Lesson-2/The-Speed-of-Sound

Umeda, N. (1977). Consonant duration in American English. *Journal of the Acoustical Society of America 61*, 846-858.

Weisstein, Eric W. (2016). Fourier Series. *In MathWorld--a Wolfram web resource*. Retrieved from http://mathworld.wolfram.com/FourierSeries.html

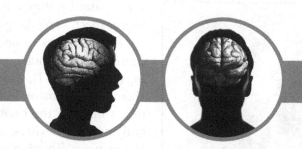

Introduction to Acoustic and Articulatory Phonetics

GOAL

Introduce the essentials of acoustic and articulatory phonetics. Examine acoustic resonance as a perceptual characteristic in the articulation and perception of speech sounds

OBJECTIVES

- Apply the functions of the major parts of a resonating system to the human vocal tract.
- Distinguish among phone, phoneme, and allophone.
- Relate vocal tract patency to phoneme articulation.
- Distinguish among the sound sources for vowels, diphthongs, approximants, plosives, and fricatives.
- Distinguish among the four major articulatory characteristics of vowels.
- Distinguish the articulatory characteristics of approximant consonants from those of nasal consonants and vowels.
- Describe or recognize any General American English vowel in terms of its International Phonetic Alphabet (IPA) classification.

• • • • • • •

THE RESONANT VOCAL TRACT

The vocal tract is an acoustic resonating system. It enables mankind to communicate by means of speech because it is uniquely capable of producing and modifying complex sound sources. By virtue of its great flexibility and its location at the distal end of the respiratory tract, the vocal tract can produce one quasiperiodic and two aperiodic sound sources and vary the spectral

Culbertson, W. R.
Fundamentals of the Speech and Language Sciences (pp 37-47).
© 2020 Taylor & Francis Group.

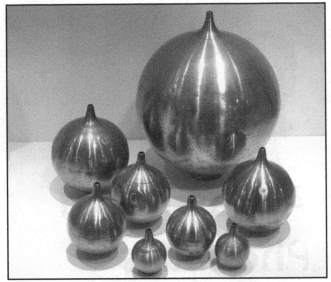

Figure 4-1. Helmholtz resonator. ("A selection of Helmholtz resonators from 1870, Hunterian Museum, Glasgow.jpg" by Stephencdickson / used under CC BY-SA 4.0 / Desaturated from original)

it emanates by amplifying some parts of the complex source spectra and dampening others.

The Helmholtz resonator consists of a large cavity connected to the outer environment by a narrow opening (see Figure 4-1). A wine bottle would make a good Helmholtz resonator. In the case of the vocal tract, you might imagine the cavity consisting of the pharynx, oral and nasal cavities, and the opening located at the lips or nares. This is a great oversimplification, as we shall see, but it is a good place to start.

Perhaps the main difference between our vocal tracts and the typical Helmholtz resonator is that our vocal tracts are so flexible. Thus, they can change their resonating properties infinitely and do so, constantly. Another important difference is that our vocal tracts have at least two resonating cavities. In this sense, the vocal tract is a double Helmholtz resonator, with two resonating cavities of variable volumes, one in front of the other, connected by a tube, also of variable volume.

RESONATING SYSTEMS

First, let's review the basics of resonating systems. As you may recall, resonating systems have two main components: a driving source and an elastic medium. The driving source provides the power to compress and rarefy the molecules in the elastic resonating medium. The vocal tract can produce three driving sources, and during speech, a speaker effortlessly produces one or a combination.

The three sources are the *phonatory* source, the *fricative* source, and the *plosive* source. Any one of the three sources can be used alone. The phonatory source is by far the most frequently employed, and can be used in combination with either other source to produce voiced obstruent consonants.

The elastic medium of the vocal tract resonating system consists of the molecules of the air in the vocal tract cavities. These cavities can be thought of as a twisted, flexible tube, closed at the glottal end and open at the lips or nares. Such a resonating system is quite familiar to acoustic physicists. It is called a Helmholtz resonator. The elastic medium of the vocal tract resonating system can create an enormous variety in the sounds

VOCAL TRACT ACOUSTICS

Phonetics is the study of speech sounds. The field of acoustic phonetics is concerned with the parameters of sound propagation associated with meaningful distinctions in speech and with the nature of speaker identification. To this end, acoustic phoneticians study the nature of speech sound sources, the changing spectra of their resonant output, and the dynamics of those changes.

For acoustic studies, the typical vocal tract may be seen as a 17-cm tube, closed at one end, extending from the glottis to the lips or, as articulatory needs present, the nares. As we have seen in the chapter on acoustics, a closed tube has predictable resonant frequency bands, depending upon the length of the tube.

Of course, 17 cm is an ideal length, and not only are individual speakers likely to have vocal tracts of differing lengths, but the vocal tract of an individual speaker will also vary slightly in length during the act of speaking. In any case, the vocal tract may be seen as a resonating system, with the driving source produced at the glottis or elsewhere, and the resonating elastic medium being the air molecules in the vocal tract's resonating cavities.

envelope of all three. It is these combinations and variations that listeners (including the speaker) receive, categorically perceive, and associate to communicate with one another.

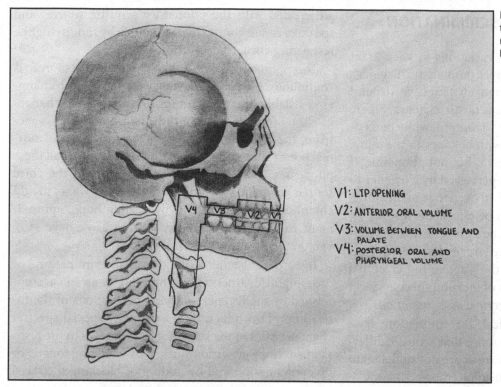

Figure 4-2. Double Helmholtz resonator as it relates to the human speech mechanism. (Image drawn by Mathew DeVore)

V1: LIP OPENING

V2: ANTERIOR ORAL VOLUME

V3: VOLUME BETWEEN TONGUE AND PALATE

V4: POSTERIOR ORAL AND PHARYNGEAL VOLUME

SOURCE AND FILTER

Meaningful speech is the product of a variable volume system by which the acoustic spectrum of a source is modified by a filter. In typical use, the filter is in constant motion, varying volumes and sources according to the speaker's demands.

The driving sources, as we have learned, are of three main types. The phonatory or glottal source is a quasiperiodic, continuous series of air pulses that pass between the vocal folds and up through the vocal tract during the open phase of the glottal cycle. The fricative source is a random, aperiodic continuous source, created by forcing a relatively laminar air flow through a tight constriction, disturbing the usual flow of respiratory air molecules and creating turbulence. The third source is the plosive source, a transient burst of energy created by trapping air behind a complete vocal tract closure and releasing it as articulatory demands require. The acoustic sources of all normal speech are one of these three, and most often variations of the phonatory, or combinations of the phonatory source and one of the other two. In the source-filter model, acoustic source spectra are referred to as *input spectra*, and those of the phonetic output are referred to as *output spectra*.

The vocal tract's resonating cavities are all located superior to the glottis, and the glottis represents the closed end of the vocal tract tube (see Figure 4-2).

These resonating cavities include the pharynx and the oral and nasal cavities. Smaller resonating cavities also play a resonating role and include the spaces between the teeth and outer tissues of the oral cavity, the small cavities of the larynx, the paranasal sinuses, and the cavity of the trachea. The larger cavities vary in volume according to the actions of the speaker to distinguish meaning in speech, while the smaller cavities help distinguish the personal identity of the speaker.

The resonating cavity volumes are crucial to phonetic variation, as they are said to filter the driving sound source. In contrast to our usual concept of a filter, this acoustic filter can either amplify or dampen the driving source, making bands of frequencies in its power spectrum louder or softer respectively. Since the speech-driving source is complex, this means that the resonating system either dampens or amplifies certain frequency bandwidths of the driving source frequency spectrum. Describing the role of the resonating system in these terms is important since two of our sources are aperiodic, and, thus, do not have discrete frequencies to amplify or dampen. It is patterns of amplification and dampening that, along with the nature of the driving source, are key perceptual features in the decoding of speech.

CATEGORICAL DISCRIMINATION

It should be apparent that variations in vocal tract acoustics can be subtle or great, and that a listener's perceptions of meaning in spoken language depend upon the magnitudes of these acoustic changes. Small, subtle acoustic changes in speech output, while perceptible, may not be associated with changes in meaning. These small changes are *phonetic*, but not phonemic. If a phonetic acoustic change is perceived by a listener to be sufficient to be associated with a change in meaning, the acoustic change is said to be *phonemic, distinctive*, or *contrastive*. It should also be apparent that perceptions of phonemic changes are largely dependent upon the linguistic background of the listener. In perceptual phonetics, the discrimination of meaningful changes in phoneme recognition is *categorical discrimination*.

Simply defined, categorical discrimination is a speaker or listener's ability to sense that acoustic differences between speech sounds are or are not sufficient to signal a change in meaning in an utterance.

A phoneme, as we have shown, is a group of speech sounds produced with similar acoustic and articulatory characteristics. Thus, a phoneme is a group of speech sounds that fall into a distinctive category by virtue of their ability to represent meaning linguistically. When differences in characteristics become sufficient, the speech sound is assigned to a different category. Listeners and speakers perceive speech sounds, or phones, as belonging to one category or another according to their acoustic and articulatory differences and, of course, the strength of categorical discriminative abilities.

SOUND SOURCES AND PHONEMES

As we have learned, one of the keys to phoneme perception and production is the nature of the driving source or sources. These sources—phonatory, fricative and plosive—are sequenced and combined in various ways to produce the sounds of any spoken language. We will limit our discussion to American English, but the same sources can be described for all languages, and some languages have even more sources.

VOWELS AND DIPHTHONGS

Vowels, diphthongs, approximants, and nasals represent the large majority of English speech sounds. All are created with the phonatory acoustic source, and speakers create contrastive variations by modifying the resonating vocal tract cavities.

The phonatory source, like the fricative source, is continuous. It frequently changes duration with changes in syllabic stress. Except for suprasegmental changes in glottal frequency, amplitude, and, sometimes, spectrum, the phonatory power source location and normal power spectrum remain unchanged across all these phonemes. In other words, the acoustics of the voice source normally vary only if the speaker wants to add emphasis or stress to the vowel, diphthong, approximant, or nasal. The aperiodic sources, as we have seen, vary in the location of their creation.

Instead, a listener's categorical discrimination, or meaningful distinction, of these phonemes is accomplished by the listener's varying perceptions of the filtered output product, rather than any special spectral characteristics of the source, itself. Changes in the resonant envelope are accomplished by changing tongue or lip configuration and by adding or blocking the nasal cavity as part of the resonating system.

VOWELS: DISTINCTIVE RESONANCE OUTPUT

Since the vocal tract is most open during the articulation of vowels, they are first in our examination of speech resonance phenomena. The phonatory source is used as the driving source for all vowels, and so, all vowels are voiced. In descriptive terms, the voicing label is considered obvious and is left unspecified.

VOWEL ARTICULATION

Vowels are articulated by changing the internal dimensions of the vocal tract tube or tubes. In fact, some speech scientists describe the vocal tract in terms of one to four tubes, taking into consideration the space in front of the tongue, the space behind the tongue, the space between the dorsum of the tongue and the roof of the oral cavity, and the space between the lips. Thus, the number of combinations is infinite and depends greatly on the phonetic environment. Changes in vocal tract tube geometry are brought about by contracting muscle groups, thereby moving the larynx, tongue, velopharyngeal sphincter, mandible, and lips.

The International Phonetic Association (IPA) classifies vowels in terms of the vocal tract configuration used to produce the specific resonance spectrum associated most with a particular vowel. Specifically, tongue position designates the location and degree of the greatest oral cavity constriction.

The location of oral cavity constriction is called the *point of maximum (or major) constriction*. The amount of patency is termed *degree of constriction*. The constriction is always in the oral cavity, but we must not forget that movements of oral structures have consequent effects on pharyngeal structures, or that the vocal tract tube resonance is affected by any changes in tube shape.

Point of maximum (or major) constriction dimensions are described as *front-central-back*. Front vowels are articulated with the tongue constricting the vocal tract near or below the superior alveolar ridge. Central vowels may be articulated with a rather neutral oral cavity constriction or with some lingual elevation near the hard palate. Back vowels are articulated with the tongue approximating the velum or posterior pharyngeal wall to varying degrees.

Degree of oral cavity (vocal tract) constriction is specified in IPA terms by close-open classification. When the tongue is low in the oral cavity, the degree is termed *open*, and when the tongue is high in the oral cavity, it is termed *close*. In between, constriction terms are said to be *mid-low, mid,* and *mid-open*. The latest IPA terminology was adopted in the mid-1990s. Before then, the terms *low* and *high* were used, respectively.

Lip-rounding constricts the vocal tract airway at its oral opening. This adds an extra constriction to the tube, and changes its resonance. It also extends the vocal tract length. In English, only the back series of vowels is associated with any degree of lip rounding, with /u/ being the most rounded. Minifie (1973) argued that lip rounding is essential as a means of fine-tuning the vocal tract in the production of back vowels.

Another characteristic of vowel articulation is the degree of muscle tension involved. Vowels may, thus, be described as *tense* or *lax*. In certain articulatory positions, vowels may be considered in tense/lax pairs, having approximately the same place and degree of vocal tract constriction and lip rounding, but different effort expended in their productions. As tenser vowels are created with higher energy, they tend to be reduced to their lax counterparts when uttered in a syllable with low stress.

Although we have used IPA terminology to describe the major characteristics of vowel articulation, we must keep in mind that the entire vocal tract resonates with the power source. This means not only the oral cavity, but also the entire pharynx.

Gunnar Fant (1970), in a landmark study done for Bell Laboratories, described the relative resonances of the oral and pharyngeal cavities during vowel articulations (see Figure 4-3). At the time, most phonetic

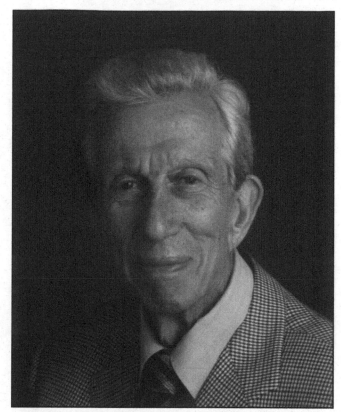

Figure 4-3. Gunnar Fant (1919–2009) helped describe vocal tract resonance. ("Gunnar Fant.jpg" by Dept of Speech Music and Hearing, KTH, Stockholm / used under CC BY-SA 3.0 / Desaturated from original)

scientists had accepted the Helmholtz resonator model of vocal tract acoustics, but most conceived a single resonating tube. Fant's findings suggested that the vocal tract is more accurately called a double Helmholtz resonator, since it has two resonating cavities: the oral cavity, and the pharyngeal cavities. Fant observed that variations in oral cavity volumes and configurations are produced by muscular forces, creating the primary resonating cavities for formants F1, F2, and F3. Formants F4, F5, and F6 are resonated more in the laryngeal cavities, not subject to nearly as much shape change. Fant would have been a two-tube scientist.

It has been known for many years that listeners categorically discriminate vowels by differentiating the sounds' spectral characteristics. Peter Ladefoged (1957), one of the seminal and ubiquitous figures in phonetic research, studied the responses of 45 English speakers of three dialect backgrounds (see Figure 4-4). He found that his listeners differentiated meaning among four vowels in minimal pair words by perceptual categorizations of the relationships of their formants within their spectral envelopes. Ladefoged also suspected that his subjects' discriminations depended on their experience

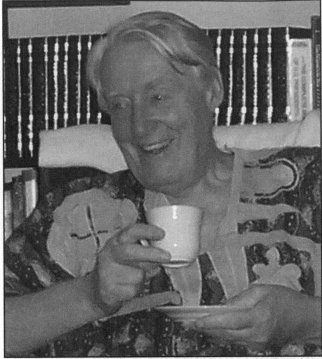

Figure 4-4. Peter Ladefoged (1925–2006) described the acoustic characteristics that underlie vowel discrimination. ("Peter Ladefoged cropped.jpg" by Pete unseth / used under CC BY-SA 4.0 / Desaturated from original)

with a given speaker's articulations of test vowels and other vowels in different contexts.

In 1952, Petersen and Barney also reported that listeners appeared to cue in to formant information in the discrimination of vowels. Since different individuals have different vocal tract dimensions and volumes, not to mention different laryngeal sources, the ratios of formant frequencies to one another, rather than the absolute values of the formant frequencies, must account for vowel discrimination. The first three formants, according to Peterson and Barney, were subject to the most change as vocal tract postures move about, and are, thus, the most crucial for the production or perception of vowel changes. Other information, such as bandwidth, amplitudes, duration, and context are important as well.

In IPA terminology, as vowels become more open, F1 increases in its center frequency. As vowels become more front, F2 center frequency increases. The fundamental is critical in its role as a driving source, but not in vowel contrast. As the fundamental frequency, F0, increases, the center frequencies of F1 and F2 will increase, but their arithmetic ratios will remain unchanged, or at least within a certain range, as long as the vowel phonemic category is not changed.

APPROXIMANTS

Approximant consonants were once referred to as *semi-vowels*. Some phoneticians cling to that label still. This is because, in a fashion similar to vowels, they are created with a relatively open vocal tract configuration, and resonance is a key feature in their perception. The fact that they also occasionally formed syllable boundaries accounted for their inclusion in the consonant category. Of course, the more closed vocal tract postures involved in approximant articulation mean that their overall amplitudes are lower than those of vowels.

Resonances of the phonatory source being vital to their perception, all approximants are voiced. All are also continuant, meaning there is no momentary speech articulator stoppage during their articulations. The English approximants are /j/, /w/, /r/, and /l/. Continuous movement is essential to the first three; in fact, they have been called glides for that reason. Momentary cessation of movement toward a vowel target during articulation of these will result in the approximant becoming a vowel, creating a diphthong with the upcoming syllabic nucleus. The lateral approximant /l/ is not considered a glide.

Much attention is generated toward blending of the American English /r/ and other pulmonic consonants. Such combinations are called *R-blends* in the lingo of applied phonetics. As one might expect, resonance characteristics of R-blends are similar to back vowels when the blending consonant is velar (such as in "fork"), and to front vowels when the blending consonant is anterior ("fort").

The only (standard) English lateral is /l/. It is produced with approximation of the lingual tip and the superior alveolar ridge, with openings created between the tongue blade and the buccal cavities on either side. With so much latitude of articulation, the lateral /l/ is heavily dependent on phonetic environment. For example, articulation of /l/ between two anterior vowels produces a light L, while articulation of the lateral posterior vowels produces a so-called dark L.

Transitions of approximant syllable releasers to their vowel nuclei are very similar to diphthong transitions. Acoustic differences are related to oral and pharyngeal volumes being more constricted in the cases of approximants, and in the fact that there is sometimes a slight degree of lip rounding observed in /r/ articulation. As mentioned above, greater vocal tract constriction results in a lower overall amplitude of the formants. Lip rounding with /r/ transitions to the vowel creates changes in F3 transition.

NASAL RESONANCE

Nasal phonemes are created by coupling the nasal cavity with the vocal tract. Nasal resonance occurs during articulation of nasal consonants, but it is also important during the articulation of vowels in a nasal phonetic environment, such as the /u/ in "moon."

Some degree of nasal resonance is considered a desirable acoustic feature of normal speech. Speech that is too nasal is called *hypernasal*, while speech without sufficient nasality is called *hyponasal*. Individuals with maxillary clefts or velopharyngeal incompetence usually have hypernasal speech, while those with nasal blockages, such as during episodes of rhinitis, may have hyponasal speech.

Nasal articulatory postures create additional space along the vocal tract. Accompanying the increased volumes are lower resonating frequencies known as *nasal murmur* and the increased presence of *anti-resonances*.

Anti-resonances are resonant frequency bands out-of-phase with the driving source. The phase discrepancy dampens the amplitudes of certain frequency bands and creates other acoustic characteristics also associated with the perception of nasality. For example, perception of nasality is related to the appearance of one or more *nasal formants*, or resonant bands created by the addition of the extra resonating cavity.

During nasal consonant articulation, the oral cavity is normally occluded, and the location of the occlusion is a major acoustic characteristic in discrimination of the phoneme. When considering nasal consonants, the importance of the place of nasal articulation in the phonemic discrimination lies in the size of the cavity created by oral cavity occlusion. When the nasal cavity is coupled with the vocal tract, and the oral cavity is closed at the place of articulation, the nasal cavity becomes the direct route of air and acoustic energy. This makes the oral cavity an ancillary resonator, the size of which depends upon where the oral cavity is closed.

In its role as a side resonator, the oral cavity is often called a *cul-de-sac* resonator (French for "Bottom of the Bag"). For nasal phonemes in most English dialects, the most anterior oral cavity closure is at the lips, thus creating the largest cul-de-sac. Articulation of the tongue and the superior alveolar ridge makes a slightly smaller cul-de-sac, nonetheless perceptible. The smallest cul-de-sac is created by articulation of the tongue back and the velum.

Anti-resonances, the energy bands out-of-phase with the driving source, appear normally in the vocal tract during running speech. They are increased in amplitude when the nasal cavity is coupled with the vocal tract, having the effect of dampening their certain formants and reducing the overall amplitude of the speech signal. Other energy bands, of course, are in-phase with the driving source and tend to amplify the signal. Energy amplification occurs at amplitude poles, while energy dampening occurs at zeros.

Nasal articulation further dampens the signal because of an increased impedance of the soft tissues found in the nasal cavity. The smaller openings provided by the nares reduces output amplitude even more.

Formant transitions are important perceptual cues with nasal articulation, just as they are in articulation of other phonemes. These transitions, from one phoneme to another, cue the listener that a nasal is present, and which nasal it is. Nasals also create a unique phonetic environment or phonetic context, having the effect of nasalizing adjacent vowels. The addition of nasal resonance to vowels that would otherwise not be nasalized is *assimilation nasality*. Assimilation nasality adds further cues for the listener about the presence of a nasal. Close vowels are more affected by nasal environment because of their increased impedance when compared with open vowels.

OBSTRUENT CONSONANTS: PLOSIVES AND FRICATIVES

The obstruent consonants are articulated by creation of a complete or nearly complete blockage of the pulmonary airstream at some point along the vocal tract. Such a blockage creates an aperiodic sound source by tapping the energy of the flowing air.

The resulting aperiodic acoustic source has a continuous spectrum, but this spectrum is modified by changing the volumes of vocal tract cavities proximal and distal to the obstruction. The result is the variation of higher peak energy levels at locations across the frequency bands of the continuous spectra.

PLOSIVES

The plosive phonemes, as their name implies, are produced with the transient aperiodic plosive source (see Figure 4-5). The sound of the plosive release is generated at the place of articulation. Its continuous power spectrum is filtered by changing the location of the source's generation and thus changing the volumes of the resonating cavities behind and in front of the place of articulation. The plosive source may be accompanied

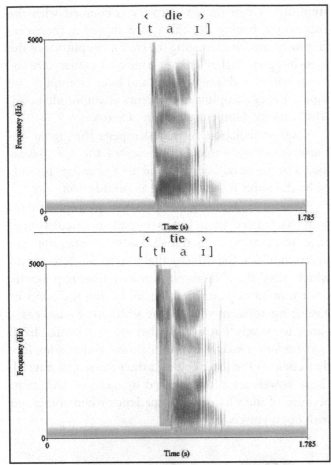

Figure 4-5. Spectrogram of words, "Die" and Tie." Note short duration of plosive source, followed by aspirated source following the plosive release for "Tie" (Bottom).

by the quasiperiodic phonatory source, with its onset generated before the release, if the plosive is voiced.

Affricates are sometimes classified as plosives with a short duration of fricative noise occurring in what is termed an *affricated release*. Any plosive can be affricated, but in English, two are strongly affricated and are called the English Affricates. These are exemplified as the syllabic boundaries of "church" and "George," /tʃ/ and /dʒ/. The IPA has not quite figured out what to do with these, so it placed them in the "Other" category of its chart.

Some plosives are not spoken with an audible plosive source. These are termed unreleased plosives or stops, and occur normally at the end of an utterance or just before a brief pause. The listener, well-acquainted with the semantics of the language, distinguishes among these plosives by perceiving ongoing acoustic resonance changes as the speaker's vocal tract transits from the previous phoneme (allophone) articulatory posture to the articulatory posture of the plosive. If the plosive

is unreleased, the plosive source will not be propagated. Instead, a period of silence will occur.

FRICATIVES

All fricatives are articulated with the fricative source, in combination with the phonatory source, as needed. The continuous, aperiodic fricative source is distinguished from the transient aperiodic plosive source by its continuous property and from the continuous phonatory source by its lack of periodicity. In this context, a continuous sound is one that can be prolonged for whatever duration the speaker desires.

As is the case with the plosive source, the power spectra of aperiodic fricative sources can vary depending upon the place of articulation at which the source is generated (see Figure 4-6). This results from varying the vocal tract cavity volumes in front of and behind the place of articulation.

SPEECH SOUND CLASSIFICATION

Since speech is a form of language based on sounds produced with the vocal tract, it is essential to study the special characteristics of the sounds. Speech sounds are used as language symbols to represent ideas, to convey information, and to evoke feelings.

The human vocal tract is a flexible air passage that, by virtue of its flexibility and the air passing through it, is suitable for making a wide variety of sounds. Shriberg and Kent (1995) estimated that one can make approximately 100 different noises with one's vocal tract. Not all these 100 noises are used as language symbols in every language, and some that are used in one language are not used in another language, or are used in a different way.

The phonemes that are used in each language and the linguistic rules for using them constitute the phonology, or sound system, of the language. As is the case for other aspects of language, users of a language tacitly accept certain linguistic rules to make communicating within that language more useful.

A phoneme is a group of speech sounds formed by similar vocal tract configurations that function as spoken language units by contrasting with other speech sound groups in a way that differentiates meaning. That means simply that changing a phoneme in speech usually results in changing the meaning of the segment.

The special characteristic that turns phones from being just any vocal tract sound into a useful member

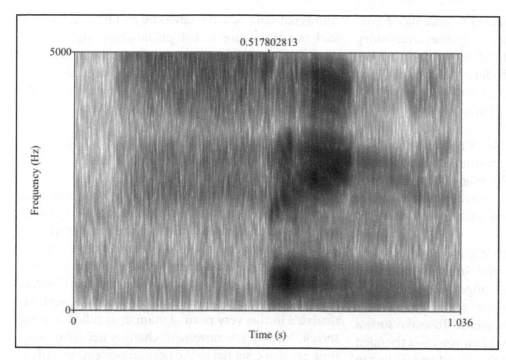

Figure 4-6. Spectrogram of the English word, "sing." Note the aperiodic fricative source beginning on the left, changing to the voiced source as the timeline continues to the right.

of a phoneme group is that the sounds are meaningful segments of speech. Vocal tract configurations may be slightly different within any phoneme group, since very few individuals can make exactly the same movements repeatedly, but the differences are not sufficient to make the acoustic result sufficiently different as to change the meaning of any word in which they are used.

Accordingly, one could argue that speech sounds used in articulating nonsense syllables are not phonemes because they have no meaning. Further, and by way of illustration, one could also argue that it is impossible to articulate a phoneme, because to do so would mean articulating all the possibilities at once. Thus, a phoneme is a conceptual entity, not a single speech sound.

When phone is associated with meaning in a spoken word, it becomes a member of a phoneme group and is termed an *allophone* of that phoneme. Minor variations in allophone articulation may be noticeable, but not sufficient to change the meanings of words in which they are spoken. When articulatory variations are sufficient to change meaning, then the phone becomes an allophone of another phoneme group.

It is conceptually useful to classify phonemes as a means of describing the phonology of any spoken language. This has been done in several ways, from simple to complex. The reason for any classification, besides a natural desire to arrange complex matters, is to better understand the dynamics of syllable articulation, with its sequential opening, closing, and juncture features.

It must be kept in mind that the study of phoneme groups has its shortcomings in application of the conceptual to the practical. Allophones are rarely uttered in isolation. Instead, they are almost always parts of a flowing stream of acoustic signals, one merging into another until the utterance is complete.

The simplest phoneme classification system would be one that specifies an open vocal tract versus a closed vocal tract. In such a binary system, any vowel, nasal, or approximant would be placed in the open vocal tract category, and any obstruent consonant would be placed in the closed vocal tract category.

The open-closed concept is at the very heart of the concept of the syllable as a sequence of articulatory postures featuring opening and closing vocal tract configurations in concert with other such postures. One might consider the syllable as a series of speech movements occurring over time, with a more closed vocal tract posture occurring at the beginning, flowing into a more open posture, and culminating with a more closed vocal tract configuration. Phonetic scientists consider the closed vocal tract configurations at the beginning and end of the syllable to be the syllable's boundaries, and the more open posture in the middle as its nucleus.

Sometimes, the boundary at the beginning of a syllable is termed its *releaser*, or it is said to be in the initial or pre-vocalic position. Likewise, the boundary at the end of a syllable is said to be its *arrestor*, or it is said to be in the final or post-vocalic position.

A speaker might be constrained to articulate a particular allophone of a phoneme by the articulatory configurations occurring just before and just after articulation of a target sound under scrutiny. This leads phonetic scientists to consider phonetic environments or phonetic contexts as an important aspect of vocal tract dynamics.

Opening and closing vocal tract postures modulate egressive pulmonary airflow, creating acoustic sources of varying amplitudes. Syllables might thus be considered pulses of acoustic energy having greater amplitudes during the open postures and lower amplitudes during the closed postures.

While the open-closed arrangement is a simple starting point, it is not very useful for much more than that. Instead, a system that arranges phonemes on a continuum, based on the degree of their open-ness or closed-ness, is much more useful. To make such a continuum, we might organize open vowels at the open end and plosive consonants at the closed end. Filling in between the two ends would be open-mid, close-mid, and close vowels, approximants, and nasals.

It is the area between the open and closed ends of the continuum where fine distinctions in spectra duration and glottal frequency are found. For example, open vowels, as their group name implies, are articulated with a more open vocal tract configuration than close vowels. The closest of the close vowels are very nearly approximants, with co-articulatory variations commonly crossing the line.

A more complex and far more widely used phoneme classification system is that of *place-manner-voicing*. Sometimes called the traditional system, it classifies phonemes according to the vocal tract location of maximum constriction, how the breath stream is managed, and the timing of any phonatory source onset during syllable articulation. Place-manner-voicing generally applies only to pulmonic consonants, with vowels described in terms of tongue position and lip rounding.

Still more complex are systems of *distinctive features*, first proposed by Jakobsen in the 1940s and refined to their most useful extent by Edwards in 2003. Distinctive feature systems apply to consonants and vowels alike, and are arrays of binary attributes felt to be phonetically contrastive (distinctive) in their presence or absence. The reality is that not all distinctive features are always distinctive, but the usefulness of the systems in further understanding articulatory dynamics is undeniable.

Distinctive feature systems and place-manner-voicing classifications help speech and language scientists describe the motor strategies used in single and connected syllable articulation by children and adults. Such strategies are called *phonotactics* and depend upon the linguistic constraints of phoneme combinations inherent in the individual's phonological system. Phonotactics strategies become more mature as speakers become more fluent in a given language.

VOCAL TRACT DYNAMICS

Up to now, we have mostly considered phonemes as singular phenomena. Of course, this is far from the reality of normal speech. Instead, the vocal tract is in almost constant motion, gliding from one posture to another posture, from open to close and open again, and, to some extent, it is this movement that conveys meaning, not to mention intent, in speech. Speech articulated in this very normal manner is called *running speech*. Vocal tract movement changes occurring over time are also essential to the normal perception and articulation of speech.

It should be apparent that normal speech is not simply combinations of individual allophones. Instead, it is more accurately viewed as a sequence of vocal tract opening and closing variations called syllables. As for speaking movements over time, it is logical to observe syllables as having beginnings, middles, and endings, and to recognize these a fundamental to a speaker's motoric images of speech flow, and also to the listener's perceptions of meaningful speech acoustics.

The movement begins as the speaker attacks the releaser or onset of the first syllable, and only stops when the speaker senses a need for a pause or a breath intake, or has finished speaking (for the time being).

Vocal tract movement, considered over time, is called *transition*, and transition is the flow from one syllable to the next. In this way, transition often results in the last syllable boundary of a preceding syllable serving as the first syllable of a following syllable. With this consideration, one might imagine that most syllable boundaries are articulated between syllable nuclei and are in medial or intervocalic phonetic environments. Such dynamic movements make running speech articulation sound "natural" to a native listener, but can confuse new learners of a language.

Phonetic scientists describe the flow of running speech from one syllable as *syllabic juncture*. When there is no pause or interval separating the end of a previous syllable from the beginning of the next syllable, the juncture is said to be closed. Closed juncture occurs most frequently in running speech. Open juncture occurs when there is an audible interval between the end of a previous syllable and the beginning or onset of a following syllable.

Transition is most readily observable in diphthong articulation, during which the vocal tract posture and resultant resonance shift from that of one vowel to that of another. It may also be observed in the articulation of certain approximants, such as /j/, /r/, and /w/. Less obvious is the importance of transition in the perception of all other phoneme combinations.

REFERENCES

Edwards, H. T. (2003). *Applied phonetics: The sounds of American English* (3rd ed.). Clifton Park, NY: Thompson Delmar Learning.

Fant, G. (1970). *Acoustical theory of speech production.* The Hague: Mouton & Co.

Jakobson, R. (1968). *Child language, aphasia and phonological universals.* The Hague: Mouton.

Ladefoged, P. (1957). Information conveyed in vowels. *The Journal of the Acoustical Society of America, 29,* 98-104.

Minifie, F. (1973). Speech Acoustics. In Minifie, F., Hixon, T., & Williams, F. (1973). *Normal aspects of speech hearing and language.* Englewood Cliffs, N.J.: Prentice Hall.

Petersen, G. E., & Barney, H. L. (1952). Control methods used in the study of vowels. *The Journal of the Acoustical Society of America, 24,* 175-184.

Shriberg, L. D., & Kent, R. D. (1995). *Clinical phonetics* (2nd Ed.). Needham Heights, MA: Allyn and Bacon.

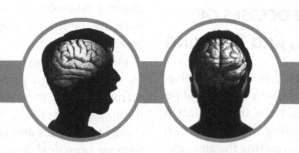

Neuroscience of Speech and Language

This chapter focuses on the neuroscience of speech. We begin with the very thoughts that occur in the speaker as the spoken communication is being contemplated, and work our way through the neurological functions required to make the acoustic signal.

The next section is a basic tour of the brain. We cover the cerebral cortex and the deep neurological centers, and their roles in creating an effective communicative utterance. We discuss the peripheral nerves that connect the brain and spinal cord to the peripheral speech mechanism.

In the third section, we cover the complex neurological systems that contribute to the smooth, voluntary motor functions necessary to create the flow of speech.

The fourth and last section focuses on neurological processes in the listener. We begin with a review of the peripheral hearing system and move through the vestibulocochlear nerve, the central auditory pathways, cerebral cortex and a brief and superficial look at psychological listening processes.

Part 1: Speech Production and Perception

GOAL

Examine the neurological processes underlying speech and listening.

OBJECTIVES

- Distinguish among communication, language, and thought.
- Compare and contrast three approaches to language development.
- Distinguish among the four levels of neurological processing events in the speaker and listener.

Culbertson, W. R.
Fundamentals of the Speech and Language Sciences (pp 49-77).
© 2020 Taylor & Francis Group.

NEUROLOGICAL PROCESSES OF THINKING, LANGUAGE, AND SPEAKING

This section covers neurological processes involved in speech. Such processes include both central and peripheral neurological processes, from the very act of deciding to speak through selecting the phonemes to build the syllables to be used, contracting the appropriate vocal tract muscles, and terminating at the mind of the listener.

At the top of the neurological hierarchy, at least in terms of complexity, would be psychological processes. Psychological processes are, after all, the products of neurological functioning. First, we will look at the relationship of thought to language, and also at speech as a language modality. After that, we will examine the cerebral anatomic centers for language expression and reception, followed by a closer look at psychological and linguistic processes of the speaker and the same processes of the listener. We must be very cursory about this, given the fact that entire courses and degree programs are based on these processes.

At the outset, we distinguish language from communication. Almost all living entities engage in some form of communication, whether it is the bright colors that attract bees to flowers, or the facial grimaces of angry mammals. This is not really language, because it does not necessarily involve thought or any symbolic mediation. It does, however, involve a complex degree of neurological functioning. Language, as treated herein, requires the even more complex neurological process of using symbols to mediate the communicative process in predictable patterns of usage.

In any case, a good place to begin our examination of a communication act would be the idea that a speaker wants to communicate something. This desire, of course, is, in itself, a psychological process, and one might imagine it would come initially in the form of a thought. Conceiving and formulating the words, or phrases or sentences that the speaker decides are best to communicate the idea also involves input and processing from multiple neurological centers, most of which are located in the brain. Just imagine the experiences, emotions, and associations that are put into play to accomplish this very early beginning to an act of communicating.

Thought can exist in the absence of language. The relationship between thought and language has been the subject of a great deal of scientific discussion for centuries. It is extremely difficult for us to contemplate thought in the absence of language, perhaps because we must use internal language to contemplate such a complex subject.

One approach may be found in the fact that, while we may use language to facilitate thought, there are many instances in which we don't need language to think. Examples of the independence of at least some thought processes and language are found in children who are born deaf. We can surely see examples of how deaf children—some of whom might be reading these very lines—can think quite well. Another example of how thoughts exist in the absence of language might be observed in adults who lose their abilities to use language through aphasia, a condition in which the language centers of the brain are damaged. Yet, individuals with aphasia seem to have only partially lost their thinking abilities.

Still, it remains extremely difficult to understand thought as it exists in the absence of language. One way to try is to consider an action immediately after you do it. Those of us who have years of experience driving automobiles, or even riding bicycles, often find ourselves arriving at our destinations without much consciousness of having piloted the vehicle. We have successfully navigated the route without having mediated the process with language. At dinner the other night, I reached over for a tortilla chip and dipped it in salsa while listening to another person talk. The action was not reflexive, being the result of the desire to obtain a chip instead of, say, a napkin. So the action clearly involved some sort of thought. But the thought was not facilitated by any internal language. I didn't say to myself, "I want a chip and salsa, rather than a napkin." Of course, immediately after I performed that action, I began to generate internal language to think about it. This also distracted my attention to my conversational partner, eliciting the usual, "Huh?" In another common example, I arrived at home one day after having driven my car several miles and listening to someone talk on the radio. While I might have been using my language skills to interpret the speech delivered through the radio during the journey, the language had nothing to do with driving, an action most would consider to involve some degree of thought.

In its purest sense, thought is an internal process by which one represents one's reality to one's self. Jerome Bruner (1966) posited that thought was manifested in terms of images, activity, and language, suggesting that language is but one aspect of thinking.

Related to the process of thinking and thought is the process of cognition. Cognition is, literally, the art of knowing. It is distinguished from language acts, although language is an important facilitator of cognition and from emotional or intuitive feelings. In other words, we can know without language, but language enables us to know some things in greater detail.

Some great cognitive psychologists of the 20th century wrote about the independence of thought and language. Jean Piaget is best known for his writings about cognitive development in children (see Figure 5.1-1). He posited several cognitive and linguistic milestones in human development that still serve as foundations for today's clinical assessments. Leo Vygotsky (1962) also distinguished between verbal and non-verbal thought, while asserting the facilitating nature of language in thought. Vygotsky emphasized that society, particularly through adult interactions, influences linguistic and, thus, cognitive development.

On the other hand, some linguists developed the notion that language reflects how we think. Benjamin Whorf is perhaps the best known of these linguists. He posited that societies develop language in terms of their cultural needs, and needs for language to facilitate these (Whorf, 1956). He cited examples, such as Eskimo words for "snow," and the theory became known to linguists as the *Whorfian hypothesis*. Current opinion has it that language may make it easier to communicate snow facts, but does nothing much to facilitate our thinking about snow.

Two aspects of language distinguish it from all other forms of animal communication. First, we can use it to create completely novel utterances: utterances that convey meaning and may have never been uttered before. We can use our linguistic rules to combine language components into products that are uniquely individual, yet can be comprehended by others who speak our language. The second aspect is that we can use language to communicate ideas about language itself. Communicating ideas about language is called *metalanguage*, and is one of the signs of advanced language ability.

Since this is a speech science course, we should focus our attention on language, particularly spoken language. A good framework upon which to contemplate the thought processes underlying spoken language is to examine the way language develops in young people (see Figure 5.1-2). There are many other approaches to this question, but a language development model provides a foundation to take into account the way thinking and communication begin and evolve.

Much has been written on language development, and much study has gone into a theoretical basis to

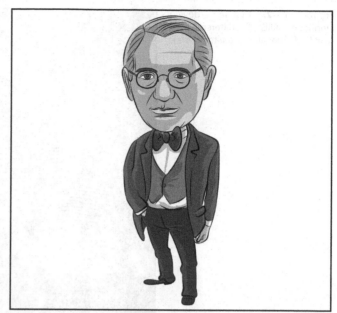

Figure 5.1-1. Jean Piaget (1896–1980) is best known for his writings about cognitive development in children. (molcay/Shutterstock.com)

describe its nature. Language is, however, probably, the most complex form of human behavior, so it is not surprising that a wide array of positions have emerged. Among those, three major viewpoints have guided study. These are the *cognitive model*, the *learning model*, and the *sociolinguistic model*.

COGNITIVE MODEL OF LANGUAGE DEVELOPMENT

The cognitive model sees language as a function of physical and neurological development. This model examines major stages in the development of thinking and in using language to mediate thinking. This was Jean Piaget's domain, although many others presented their thoughts about developmental stages. Not the least famous of these was Sigmund Freud (see Figure 5.1-3).

Although details may be slightly different among writers about developmental linguistic milestones, some major trends are of concern for those tasked with considering the need for intervention such as speech therapy in cases of delayed development. If the child is early in exhibiting target behaviors, there is no need for intervention. It is only if he or she is late that we begin to be concerned about treatment.

When examining speech behavior specifically, the first generally recognized major milestone is a stage called *babbling*. This vocal behavior appears when the child begins to play with vocalizations and phones by

Figure 5.1-2. Children develop language skills in different ways. (ESB Professional/Shutterstock.com)

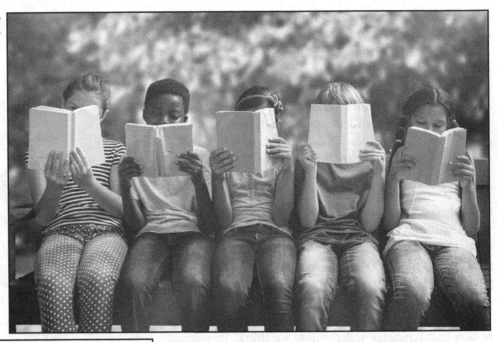

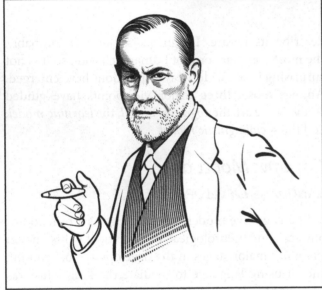

Figure 5.1-3. Sigmund Freud (1856–1939) studied the relationship of cognitive processes and language use. (Ibooo7/Shutterstock.com)

about six months of age. This vocal play is unintelligible and appears to emerge for its own sake. It is distinguished by the creation of differentiated syllables and non-syllabic utterances. At the babbling stage, one might imagine the baby is developing a phonological system to perhaps compare to that of adults and other children in the vicinity.

At the age of about one year, the child should utter her or his first meaningful words. These will usually be single-word utterances and may be approximations of the mature product. The important matter is that the child uses an intelligible utterance to stand for an idea.

The idea is called a *referent*, and the utterance is a *vocal symbol*, standing for the referent. The emergence of a first word or words suggests the early stages of a semantic system are developing.

By the child's second birthday, she or he should be combining words to form operating sentences. The sentences may be primitive, but they should be combined by some sort of linguistic rules of syntax. The child will refine these rules to closely approximate the standards of the larger population with time and experience.

Language will continue to develop in complexity as the child's nervous system and physique permit (see Figure 5.1-4). It appears that there is a critical stage of rapidly accelerated physical and neurological development, during which it is quite easy for children to "pick up" language. This period is from birth to about the age of puberty. After this stage, it becomes more difficult to learn novel linguistic rules.

LEARNING MODEL OF LANGUAGE DEVELOPMENT

Learning models of language development rely on classical and operant learning paradigms to account for language development. While the majority of clinicians have pretty well discounted a purely learning theory model of language development, learning principles certainly apply to some aspects of language development, such as word learning and syntax development. Clinicians use its principles to intervene in cases of delayed development.

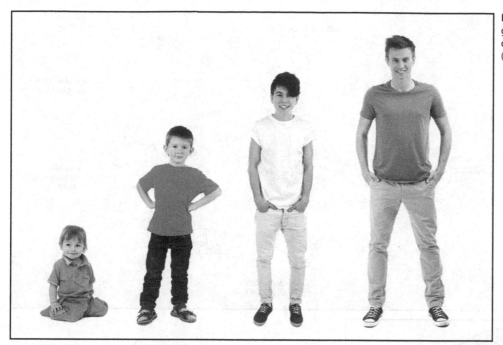

Figure 5.1-4. Speech and language development normally coincides with physical growth. (Africa Studio/Shutterstock.com)

Learning theories target a behavior that the language learner intends to learn, and then detail procedures as the learning process is consummated. The classical paradigm of learning depends on conditions that exist before the behavior occurs, and the operant paradigm depends on conditions that occur after the behavior occurs. Most language learning appears to be the result of operant learning. Language learning is reinforced by the learner getting what he or she wants after using the language properly. However, learning theorists point out that some forms of language are ends in themselves, and that language use is the end, not the means.

SOCIOLINGUISTIC MODEL OF LANGUAGE DEVELOPMENT

Sociolinguistic language development theories hold that human beings have an innate facility for language use, and that the development of language depends upon generalization of its rules in social contexts. Society and social norms play great roles in reinforcement or extinction of linguistic rules. Language rules include semantic rules, those that connect the symbol to the referent; syntactic rules, which connect the symbols to build greater language flexibility; morphological rules, which dictate changes in word structure to fit with syntactical needs; and phonological rules, which govern variations in the sounds of a language (see Figure 5.1-5).

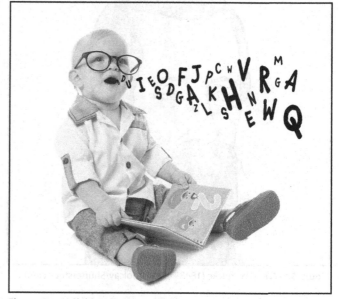

Figure 5.1-5. Children are normally born with the ability to produce the sounds of any language. (Africa Studio/Shutterstock.com)

It might be apparent, as you read this, that all these models of language development depend upon bits from the others, and that even a rudimentary understanding of language development depends on understanding all three approaches. The question often asked is, "Which principle of language development and processing is most valid?" The answer is, "All."

Whichever way one chooses to consider them, the psychological processes of speech begin with thought and the decision to create an utterance is based on thoughts or images. Other neurological processes turn those thoughts into spoken (or written, or gestured)

Figure 5.1-6. Certain areas of the cerebral cortex have been associated with specific skills, but the concept is oversimplified. (Image drawn by Mathew DeVore)

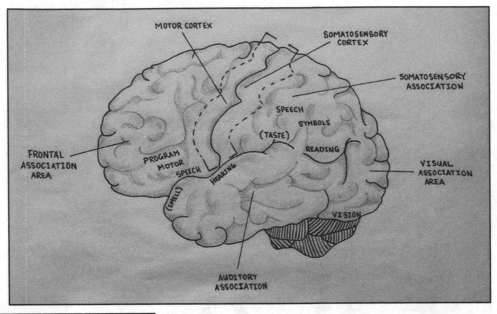

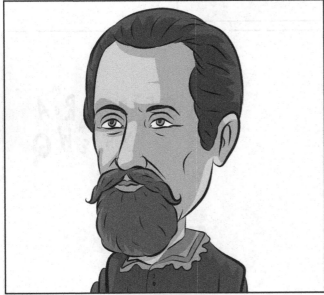

Figure 5.1-7. Karl Wernicke (1848–1905). (molcay/Shutterstock.com)

words with the intent to create images for the listener as close as possible to those conceived by the speaker.

NEUROLOGICAL PROCESSES: SPEECH PROGRAMMING AND MOTOR INNERVATION

As we said at the beginning, thoughts are products of neurological processes in the brain. Neurologists have attempted to locate specific areas of the brain for thinking, but the best that has come of those attempts is that many different centers of the brain have to work together to create thought, memory, and symbolism (see Figure 5.1-6).

The most abstract parts of spoken language seem to be functions of the thin outer layer of the cerebrum, the largest part of the brain, after processing input from all the other parts of the central nervous system. This thin outer layer is called the *cerebral cortex*.

Once the psychological or thinking processes reach the point at which ideas are to be turned into words, diffuse cerebral cortical centers feed into centers where concepts are related to mental storages of the series of articulatory postures that will combine to create speech sounds. These images apparently are stored in a speaker's memory as forms of sounds as well as sensations of muscular contractions, and even visual images of other speakers' movements. They also rely on images stored from the speaker's own sensational experiences of speaking.

There is an area of the cerebral cortex on the middle of the side of the brain, usually in the dominant hemisphere, just deep to the skin over the place where the ears emerge, at the posterior end of the lateral fissure. This area appears to be an anatomic meeting point for many of the neurons that conduct psychological processes brought into play to formulate linguistic segments. This area is sometimes called *Wernicke's area*, after Karl Wernicke, an important German neurologist (see Figure 5.1-7). Wernicke's area seems to be a very important center for the integration of diffuse cerebral images and for the association of them into one, or a series of, linguistic symbols. Wernicke's area is heavily connected by a bundle of neuronal projections called *neurites* to another cerebral area located further forward, and at the bottom of the frontal lobe.

The more forward area is called *Broca's area*, after the French neurologist, Pierre Broca (see Figure 5.1-8). Broca's area seems to be important for ordering or programming the sequences of concerted muscular motor movements required for speech. This area of the frontal lobe, usually in the dominant cerebral hemisphere, is also known as a *motor association area* because it brings forth a speaker's images of motor acts: the ideas or images of movements. Similar motor images for non-speech movements are processed in the surrounding cerebral cortex, and in the same areas of the contralateral, or opposite side, hemisphere. One must also imagine that both Wernicke's and Broca's areas must work back and forth to produce the ideas of movements that express and self-monitor the ideas of language.

Speech programming is perhaps the most complex and abstract motor act (as opposed to thinking act) in speech production. It is the ordering of the ideas of speech movement, and, while it is distinct from the decision to speak and from the selection of language elements, speech programming is largely dependent upon feedback as the movements are executed. As you can see, this process must take place between the selection of a word or phrase and the actual voluntary muscular contractions required to create the utterance of the signal.

Split-seconds after the programming of movements is accomplished, another part of the brain engages to initiate voluntary movements of the muscles of speech, located on the face, in the mouth, in the pharynx, and in the thorax. Coordination of these actions is so close that it is difficult to distinguish among them.

The part of the cerebral cortex at which vocal tract and respiratory muscles are activated voluntarily is called the *precentral* gyrus. It is located in the posterior parts of the frontal lobes of both cerebral hemispheres, just anterior to the central fissure. Here can be found the cell bodies of so-called upper motor neurons that project axons to the peripheral nerves that control the muscles of the head, neck, and thorax.

Not surprisingly, just on the other side of the central fissure is the *postcentral* gyrus, the location of the cerebral center for the reception of touch. This area allows a speaker to feel the movements of speech as one means of monitoring the utterance for accuracy.

Initiation of voluntary movement is not all that is required for smooth coordinated control of the speech muscles. Other parts of the nervous system must also engage for the effortless execution of speech movements. We will describe those parts of the central nervous system in greater detail in the next section.

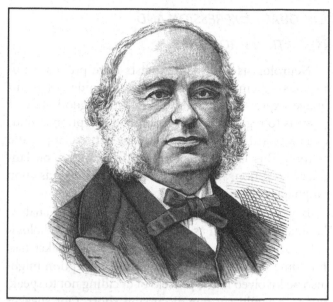

Figure 5.1-8. Pierre Paul Broca (1824–1880).

THOUGHTS IN THE LISTENER

At the other end of the communicative event is usually a listener. A listener has self-generated thoughts and images based upon unique life experiences. These might be described as well by cognitive, learning, or sociolinguistic development principles covered earlier in this chapter. It is all but certain that the listener's thoughts and images will not be identical to those of the speaker. The degree to which such images are shared by both speaker and listener is probably a function of the similarity of life's experiences, and the degree to which the speaker can formulate language that evokes the desired thoughts and images in the listener.

Interestingly, neurologists have observed tiny movements of the speech musculature occurring in the listener (Smith, Wilson, & Reisberg, 1995). These movements, called *subvocalizations*, seem to correspond to the listener's perceptions of what a speaker is saying, and suggest that the listener is using speech to enhance the experience of listening. A listener is, in this subtle way, a speaker, since the listener moves the speech mechanism in concert with the speaker in order to more completely associate and integrate the spoken message according to whatever images may exist in the memory. The speaker is also a listener to her or his own spoken utterances, and has an extra channel for receiving them: the feel of the speech mechanism as it works.

LANGUAGE EXPRESSION AND RECEPTION PROCESSES

Neurologists and psychologists have proposed numerous schemata for the processes underlying language expression and reception, but a good starting place is to regard the expression and reception as ends of a loop, with no discrete boundary between input and output. This language expression depends upon language reception, and language reception depends upon language expression.

Beginning with a speaker, then, one might analyze language expression as beginning with the psychological process of *conception*. At this stage, a speaker has, for some reason, decided to speak. Conception might also be involved in the process of deciding not to speak, but this would cut our discussion short. Our speaker has decided to speak, whether in response to some spoken input from a communicative partner, or in response to some idea occurring from memory or from the environment. In any case, the result is a thought that the speaker has decided to express.

To express the thought with spoken language, the speaker will next formulate the thought into a linguistic code, derived through the experiences of language development, likely according to one of the principles described above. *Formulation* involves the subvocal process of choosing and arranging segmental and suprasegmental phonological, semantic, and syntactic units in strings of vocal tract movements called syllables to create the appropriate acoustic signals. The syllabic sequences having been formulated, a following stage in language expression is to prepare motor images, fractions of seconds before the voluntary contractions of vocal tract muscles are to occur.

For vocal tract musculature to contract accurately and voluntarily, upper motor neurons in the frontal lobe must receive input from other brain centers. Once these upper motor neurons are activated, language expression occurs.

While spoken language expression is occurring, and, perhaps, for some period after, the speaker (it is hoped) is monitoring the act of speaking. Monitoring speech involves multiple channels of input, including audition, somesthesis (touch), and, depending upon the communicative context, vision, in much the same ways as speech input processing takes place in a listener. Vision does not contribute to speaker feedback if the speaker cannot see the listener, such as when the conversation takes place via telephone. Monitoring enables the speaker to self-correct or repair linguistic units that do not appear to be working as intended.

Language processing in the listener or communicative partner might be said to begin with reception. There are identifiable areas of the brain that physiologists have identified as being primary receptive sites for the special senses of hearing, vision, and touch. While touch might not be an important part of the listening experience, studies of subvocal movements in listeners suggest that it must play some role. If the communicative setting for a conversation is such that a listener can see the speaker, then the role of vision is obvious, as is that of hearing, whether or not the communicative partners can see one another. Reception, no matter what sense is in play, is the stage at which the brain registers that an input of hearing, vision, or touch exists.

Next the brain must sort out the input signals through perception. By drawing from memories of other inputs, perhaps similar or perhaps contrasting, the listener makes connections and comparisons of spectral, temporal, and amplitude parameters, all of which depend upon the capacities of sensory end-organs in the skin, joints, eyes, and ears.

Association of language input involves comparison of perceived signals with those stored in memory, perhaps deriving meaning or perhaps not, and storing images for future use, or discarding them as insignificant. The process of association might well trigger a response to the spoken input, and is thus continuous with that of conception. Here, one might argue, the psycholinguistic process of not responding is also one of conception, depending upon association.

REFERENCES

Bruner, J. S. (1966). *Studies in cognitive growth.* New York: Wiley & Sons.

Denes, P. B., & Pinson, E. N. (1993). *The speech chain: The physics and biology of spoken language.* New York: W.H. Freeman and Company.

Piaget, J. (1959). *Language and thought of the child.* Atlantic Highlands, N.J.: Humanities. Cited in Borden, G. J., Harris, K. S., & Raphael, L. J. (2003). *Speech science primer: Physiology, acoustics and perception of speech* (4th Ed.). Philadelphia: Lippincott, Williams and Wilkins.

Smith, J. D., Wilson, M., & Reisberg, D. (1995). The role of subvocalization in auditory imagery. *Neuropsychologia, 33,* 1433-1454.

Vygotsky, L. S. (1962). *Thought and language.* Cambridge, MA., M.I.T. Press. Cited in Borden, G. J., Harris, K. S., & Raphael, L. J. (2003). Cited in *Speech science primer: Physiology, acoustics and perception of speech* (4th Ed.). Philadelphia: Lippincott, Williams and Wilkins.

Whorf, B.L. (1956). *Language, thought and reality.* Cambridge, MA., M.I.T. Press. Cited in Borden, G. J., Harris, K. S., & Raphael, L. J. (2003). *Speech Science Primer: Physiology, Acoustics and Perception of Speech,* (4th Ed.). Philadelphia: Lippincott, Williams and Wilkins.

Part 2: Cortical Centers for Language Production and Perception

GOAL

Examine the form and function of major nervous system structures involved in speech and language.

OBJECTIVES

○ Describe the general organization of the human nervous system.
○ Describe the gross anatomy of the brain.
○ Describe the differences in dominant and non-dominant hemispheres.
○ Identify two communicative functions each of the frontal, parietal, occipital, and temporal lobes.
○ Relate the general roles of subcortical centers to communication.

• • • • • • •

THE HUMAN NERVOUS SYSTEM

The human nervous system is the major means by which the human body communicates within itself and with the outer environment. It is usually said to have two main divisions: a *central division* and a *peripheral division*. The distinctions between the two divisions are often described in both functional and structural terms, although some parts overlap.

The central division is said to consist of the brain and spinal cord, and in this section, we focus our attention on the outer layer of the brain tissue, called the cerebral cortex. The peripheral division is usually considered to consist of the cranial and spinal nerves and the autonomic nervous system.

It is in the brain of the speaker that the intent to speak occurs and subsequent neurological processes create the coordinated interactions of systems that produce the sounds of speech. A simple model of this process would include conception of the idea to be conveyed through speech, including the intent to speak; the formulation of the sequences of symbols to mediate the thought transmission, including the selection of symbols and their order; the voluntary activation of muscular contractions required to express the sounds of speech; and the monitoring of speech sounds and tactile feedback by the speaker to ensure the desired effect.

In the brain of the listener, acoustic symbols are received, perceived, sorted out, and associated with stored images interpreted and processed as needed.

THE CENTRAL NERVOUS SYSTEM

Anatomically, the central nervous system is composed of the brain and the spinal cord. Essentially, it is a mass of neurons and their neurite fibers embedded in a matrix of connective tissue and coated in three layers of nutritive and protective tissue. It is contained in and protected by the bones of the cranium and spinal column.

Without the peripheral nervous system, the brain is ineffective. Functionally, the central nervous system is a mediator between the receptors and effectors of the peripheral nervous system. The central nervous system depends upon input from and output to the peripheral nervous system. Input comes in the form of sensations, many of which are delivered ultimately through the spinal cord and brain stem to higher levels of the brain. Output is transmitted from higher brain levels through the brain stem and spinal cord and, ultimately, through glands and muscles. With these assets, the brain controls cognitive and sensorimotor functions.

In this section, however, we will focus on the structure and function of the brain as it applies to speech and language, because speech and language is a major modality of that mediational function attributed to the central nervous system. We have spent a lot of time evolving and developing the brain, and we probably have a long way to go.

General Structure of the Brain

The brain is composed of similar halves called *hemispheres*, with two *cerebral hemispheres* and two smaller *cerebellar hemispheres*. The cerebellar hemispheres are located below and toward the back of the cerebral hemispheres. A great number of interconnecting nerve fiber bundles called *tracts* allow the diffuse parts of the hemispheres to communicate. The cerebral and cerebellar hemispheres are separated superficially by large fissures, but interconnect deep within these fissures.

The entire brain functions as a whole to allow human beings to function at their highest levels, including acts of communicating. In general, the cerebral hemispheres process internal and external input to create the most complex psychological functions comprising the personality, while the cerebellum unconsciously processes complex movements as directed by the cerebrum.

A distinct central structure of the cerebral hemispheres, composed of the thalamus and hypothalamus, allows initial processing of information originating within and outside the body, and a brain stem serves as a collection and unconscious refinement center for the brain's mediational impulses.

On a tissue level, our brains are made up of a vast array of neurons, supported by neuroglia. Groups of neuron cell bodies in the cerebral cortex and elsewhere are usually seen as *gray matter*, due to their color, while neurite projections from the cell bodies converge in tracts called *white matter*, due to their off-white color. White matter tissue forms the main connections between brain centers and is the largest physical part of the brain. In general, gray matter does the deep slow thinking and processing, while white matter conducts fast transmission of action potentials from one set of gray matter cell bodies to another.

Cerebral Hemispheres

The two cerebral hemispheres are the most obvious parts of the brain. Visually and anatomically, they are mirror images of each other, although one is usually a bit larger. Each cerebral hemisphere is composed of several layers. The most superficial layer is the thin cerebral cortex. Deep into that is an intermediate layer of white matter that conveys neural information among other cerebral centers and the cortex. Deep to this white matter are gray matter neuron centers called nuclei, usually referred to as *subcortical* structures.

The thickness of the cerebral cortex ranges from 1.5 to 4.5 mm (0.06 to 0.18 inches). The tissue of the cortex is wrinkled, allowing it to crowd more thinking cells (neurons) into the cranial cavity of the skull. The wrinkles are called *convolutions*. The parts of a convolution one can see on superficial examination are *gyri* (singular: *gyrus*), and the parts not so readily visible are *sulci* (singular: *sulcus*). A particularly important or large sulcus is called a *fissure*.

Gyri and sulci have particular names based on their locations. For example, the largest sulcus is the one that separates the cerebral hemispheres, and it is called the *interhemispheric* or *longitudinal fissure*. The fissures located roughly in the centers of each hemisphere are the *central fissures*. The gyri in front of each central fissure are the *precentral gyri*, and the ones behind each central fissure are the *postcentral gyri*.

The neurons of the cerebral cortex must interconnect in order to perform their main processing functions. Some are connected by large nerve fiber bundles called tracts. Tracts have long axons projecting up and down to and from subcortical centers and beyond, all the way down to the lower spinal cord. Other tracts project across and between the cerebral hemispheres. Neurons located close to one another have short connections between them. Some cortical neurons have short axons to communicate with other cells in the same region

Neurons of the cerebral cortex receive input from and project output to various regions. One of these is the *thalamus*, the main relay center for all sensory input except the sense of smell. Other input to a cerebral hemisphere comes from the opposite (contralateral) hemisphere, and, of course, adjacent centers in the same hemisphere.

Functional Centers of the Cerebral Cortex

It seems apparent that the brain functions best as a holistic entity, with all its parts orchestrated to work toward a unified end. However, specific areas of the cortex have been associated with specific functions. These areas were first identified by comparing autopsy examinations with observations of an individual's behavior during life. In 1909, Korbinian Brodmann (see Figure 5.2-1) used microscopic examination to discover unique structural differences in the neurons and the strata of neutron distribution of certain cerebral cortical areas (Garey, 1999). He identified 52 areas, some with distinct borders and others with more vague borders, and gave them numbers. He did not, however, assign specific functions to these areas, leaving that to some who wrote earlier and others who wrote later, but he did compare similar areas in human brains and those of other species. His numbering system is still used today by many anatomists (see Figure 5.2-2).

Lobes of the Cerebral Cortex

The cortex of each of the cerebral hemispheres is divided by several distinct sulci, and the areas between these major sulci are called *lobes*. There are four lobes for each hemisphere, and these are called *frontal*, *parietal*, *temporal*, and *occipital* lobes, depending upon the bones of the skull cap, or *calvaria*, under which they lie.

Bearing in mind that the brain functions best in concert, physiologists have attributed functional roles to areas within the cortical lobes. These functions may be described as primary areas, for which a specific receptive or expressive function may be attributed, or association areas, which appear to be meeting points for processing input from other cerebral areas. We will examine a few of them here.

Frontal Lobe

The primary functions of the frontal lobe appear to be motor and affective or intellectual. Thus, there are many communicative functions associated with the frontal lobe. Functional centers located in the frontal lobe are often associated with speech output, and these are called *anterior centers*.

The frontal lobe is separated from the parietal lobe by a central fissure. The gyrus just in front of the central fissure is thus named the precentral gyrus, and is also sometimes called, simply, the motor cortex, Brodmann numbered this gyrus Area #4, and a similar area, the paracentral gyrus, just anterior, as Area #6. As mentioned earlier, these areas are the locations for the cell bodies of neurons whose functions are to initiate voluntary movement and to suppress involuntary movement of the head, neck, trunk, and extremities.

Communicative functions of these tracts are readily apparent. Assuming most communication is voluntary, muscular contractions necessary for facial expression, head gestures, vocal tract articulation, voluntary extremity movements, and many others are essential to all modalities of human communication.

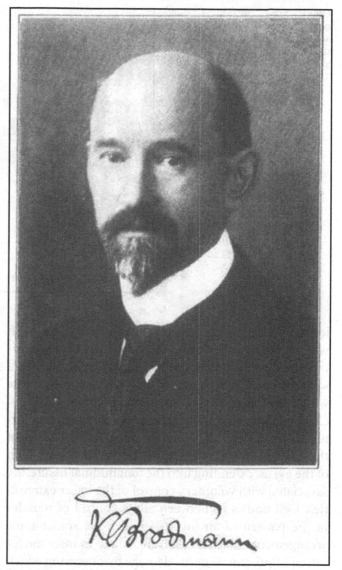

Figure 5.2-1. Korbinian Brodmann (1868–1918).

The nerve tracts that project from cell bodies in the precentral and paracentral gyri are called the *pyramidal tracts*. They enable a speaker to voluntarily contract the muscles of the vocal tract and respiratory system, not to mention skeletal muscles in the rest of the body, and also enable the speaker to suppress involuntary contractions, such as the natural tendency of a voluntary muscle to resist being stretched by an opposing muscle or by gravity. Damage to these cell bodies, or to the axon tracts that project from them, results in the inability to initiate voluntary muscular contractions and the inability to inhibit reflexive contractions such as the muscle stretch reflex.

Interestingly, extensive study of the precentral gyrus has revealed a somatotopic arrangement of the cells of the pyramidal tract. That is, cell bodies in specific

Figure 5.2-2. Brodmann distinguished areas of the cerebral cortex according to differences in their cell structures. ("1307 Brodmann Areas. jpg" by OpenStax / used under CC BY 4.0 / Desaturated from original)

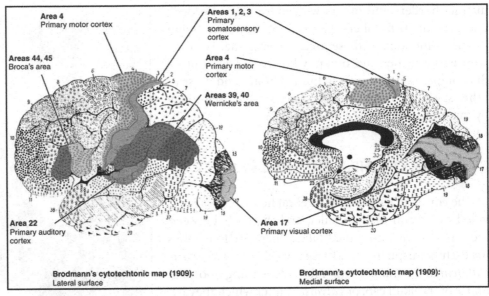

Area 4
Primary motor cortex

Areas 1, 2, 3
Primary somatosensory cortex

Areas 44, 45
Broca's area

Area 4
Primary motor cortex

Areas 39, 40
Wernicke's area

Area 22
Primary auditory cortex

Area 17
Primary visual cortex

Brodmann's cytotechtonic map (1909):
Lateral surface

Brodmann's cytotechtonic map (1909):
Medial surface

locations along the precentral gyrus are associated with voluntary control of specific body areas corresponding to the somites that underlie the ultimate body wall structure of a developing fetus, on the opposite side with a few exceptions in cranial and cervical regions. Cell bodies located at the inferior end of the motor cortex are associated with voluntary control of muscles of the head and neck, while those of the superior region of the gyrus, extending into the longitudinal fissure, are associated with voluntary control of the lower extremities. Cell bodies in between allow control of muscles in the pattern of an inverted body. The somatotopic arrangement makes it relatively simple to infer the location of precentral gyrus damage by observing which muscles are paralyzed.

Neurons comprising most of the pyramidal tracts project their axons to muscles on the opposite side of the body. The result is that neurons of the motor cortex on the left hemisphere control voluntary contractions and relaxations of muscles on the right side of the body, and vice versa. There are a few exceptions to this situation, and they involve muscles of the head and neck, including some in the vocal tract.

Another frontal lobe area of interest to speech and language scientists lies just below and in front of the precentral gyrus. This association area is called *pars triangularis* (triangular part) because it resembles a rounded triangle. Brodmann identified two kinds of neurons in this area, and numbered them Areas #44 and #45. Neurons in the pars triangularis may be considered a motor association area for movements of head and neck musculature, particularly speech muscles. These motor association area neurons pre-plan

complex, sequential voluntary movements. In the dominant hemisphere, this area is called Broca's area, after Pierre Paul Broca, the French anatomist.

Broca discovered that lesions in this area affect a patient's ability to plan the movements of speech, even though that person could still contract the same muscles reflexively or unintentionally. Other motor association areas of the frontal lobe cortex project to the extremities, and function in formulation of complex movements involving muscles of the arms, hands, legs, and feet. Individuals who have injuries to these cortical areas have great difficulty executing programmed movements such as the sequential movements of the vocal tract. Such conditions are called *apraxia*, and are distinguished from speech disorders that result from the inability to move muscles or those that involve selection of phoneme patterns.

Since frontal cortex motor association areas appear to play roles in the thoughts or images of movements, some (Bak et al., 2001) have speculated that these areas are also fundamental to the recall of verbs in speech. In support of this idea is the fact that motor association areas of the frontal lobe cortex are directly connected to those of the parietal and temporal lobes.

At the very front of the frontal lobe is the prefrontal cortex. It is associated with complex personality functions, such as affect, memory, and emotion. Brodmann numbered the prefrontal cortex Areas #9, #10, #11, and #12. This cortical area is a meeting point for association nerve fiber tracts from other cerebral cortical areas and for tracts emanating from the subcortical hypothalamus (Ojemann & Mateer, 1979). Damage to these

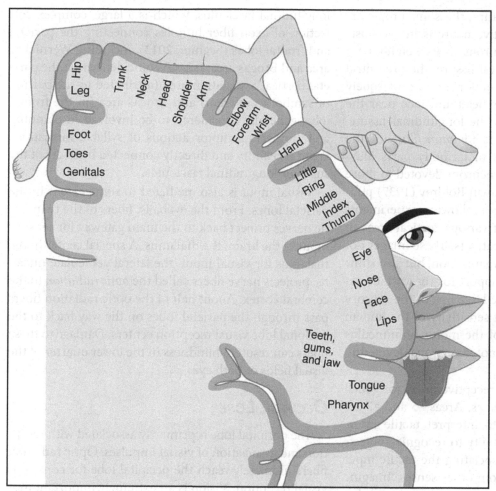

Figure 5.2-3. Sensory Homunculus. ("1421 Sensory Homunculus.jpg" by OpenStax College / used under CC BY 3.0 / Desaturated from original)

areas impacts affective behavior, including memory and emotion.

The role of voluntary vocal tract motor function for the relatively effortless planning and execution of speech movements should be clear. Not as clear, perhaps, might be the role of affective psychological functions involving personality, intent and memory in communication between human beings. When one considers that pragmatic aspects of communication involve the initiation or response to conversation, the maintenance or appropriate shifting of topics, and the termination of the communicative act, the role of the anterior frontal cortical neurons in pragmatic interpersonal communication becomes more apparent.

PARIETAL LOBE

The parietal lobe is generally associated with tactile reception and interpretation. The tactile sense includes the awareness of physical contact as well as the sensation of position and movement. Other parietal areas play roles in the images involving the tactile sense.

Located just posterior to the frontal lobe, on the posterior side of the central sulcus, the parietal lobe includes the postcentral gyrus, the primary receptive site for conscious tactile reception. In this gyrus are neurons that receive neural impulses generated by touch stimuli of various types and bring them into consciousness to the individual. The postcentral gyrus is sometimes called the *somesthetic cortex* because it brings awareness to feelings delivered to the body wall.

Brodmann identified four structurally different areas of the postcentral gyrus, and numbered them, from anterior to posterior, Areas #3, #1, and #2, plus a small area located at the inferior end of the central sulcus which he numbered Area #43. These areas have been generally attributed with various stages of tactile reception. Neurons of the postcentral gyrus are arranged somatotopically, and correspond to the motor strip in somatotopic representation (see Figure 5.2-3). They serve, generally, the function of bringing sensations of pain, temperature, gross touch, vibratory sense, and proprioception to consciousness.

Many images exist illustrating the somatotopic arrangement of sensory receptive neurons in the postcentral gyrus and motor neurons in its neighbor on the opposite side of the central fissure, the precentral gyrus. These generally take the form of a grotesquely shaped individual, having its head and face near the lateral fissure and its feet in the longitudinal fissure. Such an image is referred to as a *homunculus*, and the disproportionate dimensions of its body parts illustrate the varying numbers of neurons devoted to those parts. Wilder Penfield and Edwin Boldrey (1937) published the first of these images following experiments with electrical stimulation of various cortical areas in locally anesthetized human patients. These images not only show the somatotopic organization, but also show the degree of neurological support for the various somatic areas. For example, the large lips in the sensory homunculus reflect the great sensitivity of the human lips, while the large hands of the motor homunculus reflect the great number of motor neurons devoted to fine finger control.

Adjacent to the primary receptive areas for touch are the parietal association areas. Areas #5 and #7 are associated with the ability to interpret tactile information. *Stereognosis* is the ability to recognize objects by feeling them, perhaps associating the tactile input with previous stimulation from other senses. Imagine identifying the difference between a quarter and a key in your trouser pocket without seeing either one. One might also imagine that monitoring and planning movements, such as those of speech, facial, and other gestures, not to mention handwriting, would be at least partially mediated by associative parietal functions, including the reception, perception, and images of tactile impressions.

Perhaps the most complex association cortex is Wernicke's area. The location of Wernicke's area is disputed by some, but most, including this writer, consider it to lie not only in the parietal lobe, but to spread over to include parts of the posterior temporal lobe as well. Brodmann's Areas #39 and #40, the angular gyrus and supramarginal gyrus, respectively, comprise Wernicke's area. Neurolinguists sometimes refer to these parts of the cerebral cortex as posterior areas.

Association of auditory (supramarginal) and visual (angular) symbols with their referents appears to be least partially mediated here, particularly in the dominant hemisphere. Located posterior to the end of the lateral fissure, in the cortical juncture of the parietal and temporal lobes, these areas are heavily connected to the frontal motor association areas by the superior longitudinal fasciculus, which is a large, complex collection of axon fiber bundles connecting the parietal and frontal lobes (Seghier, 2013), including Wernicke's area and Broca's area. It is no coincidence that the parietal cortical association area (attributed to the pairing of symbol to referent) and Broca's area (in the frontal lobe, generally considered to be involved in planning and connecting motor actions of syllable formation) are in proximity and directly connected by fibers of the superior longitudinal fasciculus.

Visual input is also mediated to some extent in the parietal lobes. From the eyeballs, fibers of the twin optic nerves project back to the main gateway for sensory input in the brain, the thalamus. A special center in the thalamus for visual input, the lateral geniculate nucleus, projects nerve fibers called the *optic radiation* to the cerebral cortex. About half of the optic radiation fibers pass through the parietal lobes on the way back to the occipital lobe visual reception centers. Damage to these fibers can result in blindness in the lower quarter of the visual fields of both eyes.

OCCIPITAL LOBE

The occipital lobe is primarily associated with reception and association of visual impulses. Optic radiation fibers ultimately reach the occipital lobe for conscious visual reception. Vision is an extremely important modality for communication in human beings, particularly considering that we are the only beings known to read and write.

The occipital lobe is located in the posterior portion of the brain, deep to the occipital bone. The parieto-occipital fissure, clearly visible by examining the medial surfaces of the hemispheres, separates the occipital lobe from the parietal lobe. It is difficult to distinguish the borders of the occipital lobe by examining the brain's lateral surface, but if one examines the cortex within the longitudinal fissure, it is easy to see the line between the parietal lobe and the occipital lobe. The physical boundary between occipital and temporal lobes is not very distinct. This is, perhaps, an anatomic testament to the interplay of visual and auditory, not to mention tactile, signal processing.

The primary cortical receptive area for conscious visual input is located within the calcarine sulcus, medial and inferior to the parieto-occipital sulcus. This is Brodmann's Area #17, and it is here that the brain first registers the existence of conscious visual images. Since the receptive neuron cell bodies are contained in the two walls lining the calcarine sulcus, they can be organized into at least four distinct regions, one for each wall of the fissure for each hemisphere. In this way, central projection of the visual field is organized into roughly four quadrants for each eye, merged through perceptual environmental experiences.

Damage to the visual receptive centers in the calcarine sulcus causes various degrees of cortical blindness. In such cases, the peripheral visual system may be perfectly healthy, but the affected individual registers no consciousness of visual input. There may even be a pupillary response to concentrated light, but no awareness of the light's presence. Lack of visual consciousness may also be a function of damage or dysfunction of adjacent visual cortical areas involved in perception or even association. It is a diagnostic problem of import to professionals working in several fields of the health professions.

Optic nerve fibers originate in special sensory cells located in the retina of each eye. Fibers projecting from these special cells aggregate at the rear of the eye to form the paired optic nerves. The optic nerves carry light generated nerve impulses from the eyes back to the brain, where they are received consciously or unconsciously. Those impulses destined to create conscious light reception pass through the lateral geniculate nucleus of the thalamus and ultimately arrive at the calcarine sulcus. Other nerve impulses destined to create unconscious, reflexive responses, such as pupillary constriction, arrive at special centers in the brain stem.

Before stimulating the retinal sensory cells, light energy must pass through the cornea and lens of each eye, and, since light energy travels in a straight line, the energy from the visual field is projected upside down and backwards. In addition, there are normally two images being sent to each occipital lobe, one from each eye. This seemingly confusing arrangement is ultimately sorted out by processing in association cortical areas surrounding the primary visual receptive areas in the calcarine sulcus so that a person is unaware of the dual upside-down and backwards arrangement.

Perception and association of visual images is a function of neurons in the association cortex adjacent to visual receptive areas. There are many levels of visual perception, including color perception, depth perception, and various degrees of image discrimination. Recognition of a visual stimulus is accomplished by comparing it with other items in memory. Progressively more complex levels of association occur by recruiting neuron pools in other brain areas. For example, reading involves input from auditory cortex, while writing must also bring tactile association and fine motor skills into play.

Vision plays a fundamental role in interpersonal communication at many levels. The role of vision in graphic communication is obvious, but vision plays a crucial role in simple spoken communication, as well. In simple conversations between individuals, face-to-face interaction involves more than just the sounds of speech. Most of us look at the faces and even oral movements of those with whom we speak, often to the point of mimicking those movements. To appreciate how much we rely on vision during simple interpersonal conversations, think of the development and role played by emoji images to help convey feelings in telephone text or email messages.

TEMPORAL LOBE

The last of the cerebral cortex lobes is the paired temporal lobes. Located inferior to the frontal and parietal lobes, anterior to the occipital lobes, and inferior to the lateral sulcus, the temporal lobes occupy most of the inferior part of the cranial cavity's middle fossae.

Temporal lobe functions are, in some ways, difficult to separate from the other brain functions. This is because a major function of the temporal lobes seems to be to coordinate functions of the other parts of the brain. Neurons in the temporal lobes have many intercortical connections, and all its functions are not yet clear.

There are three temporal lobe gyri, called, appropriately enough, the superior, middle, and inferior gyri. At the posterior end of the superior temporal gyri and straddling the opercular part of that gyrus on either side is an area called *Heschl's gyrus*. This is a cortical area of great interest to audiologists and speech-language pathologists, because it is the primary receptive site for sound generated action potentials arriving from the cochleae. Brodmann numbered this site #41 and #42.

Just as is the case for vision and any other special sensory input, there are progressively more complex levels of auditory processing. These are functions of the central auditory system.

At the most basic level is *sensation*. This is nothing more than the awareness of the existence of a stimulus. To be sensed, or brought into consciousness, the stimulus has to have sufficient intensity to trigger action potentials. Thus, sensation is dependent upon the condition of the peripheral hearing system.

After an auditory stimulus has become conscious, a listener must distinguish it from other auditory signals through the process of *perception*. Perception can be summarized in terms of distinguishing the characteristics of the stimulus. As we learned in the chapter on acoustics, acoustic characteristics include frequency, amplitude, and spectrum. These are perceived as pitch, loudness, and quality, respectively.

Psychologists have described various levels and types of perception, and these have been subjects of many scientific studies over many years. For example, *auditory discrimination* is the ability to determine differences between similar auditory signals, such as a bell and a chime, or two periodic tones of nearly the same frequency. *Speech discrimination* is the ability to distinguish between similar sounding words, such as "goat" and "coat." *Figure-ground discrimination* is the ability to distinguish an auditory signal from background noise, and, as we learned in the chapter on acoustics, is largely dependent on signal-to-noise ratio.

Perhaps the highest level of sensory processing is association. As their names imply, association areas of the cerebral cortex are diverse, and generally extend away from a primary site towards other cortical sites. The neurons of association areas bring into play functions of the rest of the cerebral hemispheres in the processing of certain stimuli. In addition to the short fibers facilitating communication among neurons in adjacent areas of the cerebral cortex, many long neural fiber bundles connect distant areas within and between the cerebral hemispheres. These long bundles are called *fasciculi* (singular: *fasciculus*), a Latin word meaning a bundle of fibers.

For auditory stimuli, one can imagine a listener might associate auditory input with visual, tactile, and even motor functions, particularly when it comes to the processing of spoken language. Although some sources designate Brodmann's Area #22 as the site for auditory association (e.g., Karbe et al., 1995), this is far too simple an explanation. At the association level of sensory processing, some sort of meaning or relationship is attached to the input, involving multiple areas of the cerebral cortex, depending upon the nature and complexity of the stimulus, and including, as you may have already speculated, input from memory.

The temporal lobe also plays a role in visual image processing in the same way as the parietal lobe. On the way back to the occipital lobe, optic radiation fibers from the lateral geniculate nuclei of the thalamus deviate through the temporal lobe in a tract known as *Meyer's loop*. These tracts convey neural impulses associated with visual information originating in the inferior halves of each retina back to the occipital lobe.

Some studies have associated Meyer's loop fibers with language functions, particularly language lateralization, as a bundle of the arcuate fasciculus (Nowell et al., 2016; Sreedharan et al., 2015).

CEREBRAL DOMINANCE

One of the cerebral hemispheres is called the *dominant hemisphere*. For the vast majority of individuals, but not all, this means the left cerebral hemisphere. Some are right-hemisphere dominant, and others have mixed dominance. Dominant is, perhaps, a misleading term if taken to imply that one hemisphere dominates or suppresses the functions of the other. Such is not the case, however, as each hemisphere has its own necessary contribution.

In most individuals, however, there is a functional asymmetry between the two hemispheres. One example of this is manifested in language functions of the hemispheres. The dominant hemisphere of most individuals seems to be the functional seat of segmental language functions such as semantic meaning, syntactical rules, and phonological processes, while the non-dominant hemisphere seems to serve more non-segmental functions, such as speech intonation, tempo, and pauses. In fact, the terms Wernicke's area and, Broca's area typically apply only to those cortical regions in the dominant hemisphere, and it is rare for individuals having non-dominant hemisphere brain damage to suffer from *aphasia*, a disruption of segmental language functions resulting from damage to the cerebral cortex.

For many years, it was assumed that since most people are right-handed, and most people are left-hemisphere dominant, and since the motor cortex of the left hemisphere controls voluntary contractions of the muscles on the right side of the body, there must be some relationship between handedness and cerebral dominance. According to that supposition, all right-handed people are left-hemisphere dominant, and all left-handed people are right-hemisphere dominant.

This supposition turns out to have little support. In 1998, Willard Zemlin reported a historical summary of many studies regarding the relationship between handedness and cerebral dominance. He noted that in studies of right-handed subjects, 90% were left hemisphere dominant, while in studies of left-handed subjects, 64% were also left hemisphere dominant. In other studies, focusing on right hemisphere dominant subjects, only 20% were left-handed.

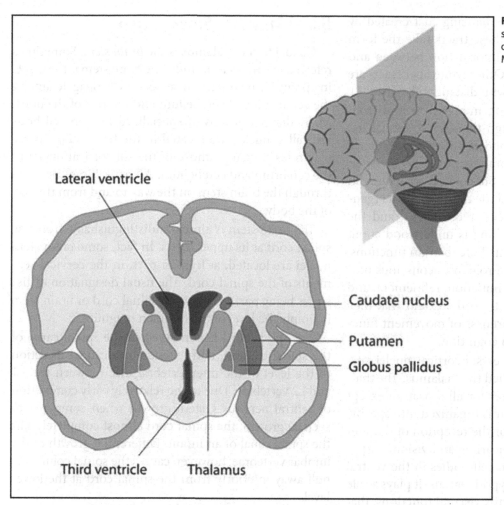

Figure 5.2-4. Subcortical cerebral structures such as the basal nuclei can be seen in a coronal section. (Alila Medical Media/Shutterstock.com)

One problem with studies of this issue is the method for determining cerebral dominance. Historically, the most reliable way was to examine the case histories of individuals who were affected by aphasia. In more recent years, a *Wada* test (Wada, 1997) has been performed, during which a brain function–inhibiting chemical is injected into either the right or left internal carotid artery to observe its effect on cognitive functioning.

A less invasive and less risky method of determining cerebral dominance is *functional transcranial Doppler measurement*. In this procedure, sensitive ultrasonic equipment is used to compare the rate of blood flow to each hemisphere and observe any changes or asymmetries in subjects performing a wide variety of cognitive tasks, including language (Connaughton, Amiruddin, Clunies-Ross, French, & Fox, 2017).

SUBCORTICAL BRAIN STRUCTURES

The cerebral cortex does not function alone. As important to language and other forms of communication as it is, brain structures deep in the cerebral hemispheres, in the paired hemispheres of the cerebellum, in the brain stem, and in the spinal cord provide important infrastructure without which the cerebral cortex would have no value. These centers consist mainly of neuron cell body groups having special properties that allow the cerebral cortex to perform its conscious voluntary functions smoothly and in concert with the rest of the nervous system (see Figure 5.2-4).

Providing pathways by which the cell body groups can communicate are white fiber tracts, similar to those we described in the cerebral hemispheres. The tracts are white in color because of the presence of myelin, an insulating and stimulus-enhancing coat created by certain glial cells. Some of these tracts take the form of loops, circulating neural information between and among all the brain centers. Other white fiber tracts are long and connect the brain with distant body parts.

Ascending and descending impulses to and from the hemispheres pass through the several specialized collections of neuron cell bodies called *nuclei*. Since these are deep to the cerebral cortex, they are often called *subcortical structures*. Subcortical structures in the cerebral hemispheres include the basal nuclei (ganglia), the subthalamic nucleus, red nucleus, and the substantia nigra. Not everything is understood about these bodies and all they contribute to brain functions, but they are known to play a role in unconscious motor functions, including the initiation, refinement, and cessation of gross movement. To the extent that they underlie an individual's awareness of movement functions, they also play a role in cognition.

The basal nuclei and other subcortical nuclei surround a central structure called the thalamus. The thalamus is the main relay center for all sensation except the sense of smell. As such, it is organized into specific groups of cells specialized for the reception of the specific senses of touch, taste, hearing, and vision. A specialized collection of neuron cell bodies in the ventral part of the thalamus is the hypothalamus. It plays a role in the integration of the body's visceral functions, that is, those associated with the internal organs, and the body's somatic functions, associated with the muscles, integument, and other support structures of the body wall.

CEREBELLUM

Occupying the posterior and lower spaces of the cranium are the twin hemispheres of the cerebellum. These lie dorsal to the brain stem and have large connections to it and, subsequently, the cerebrum. The cerebellum is anatomically similar to the cerebrum, having an outer layer of cerebellar cortex, interconnecting white myelinated fibers, and subcortical nuclei. It plays a major role in the important functions of unconscious proprioception underlying coordinated movement and motor learning. Here, as is the case with the cerebrum, the cerebellum contains many loops of interconnecting fibers, conveying neural information to and from the cerebrum and distant areas of the spinal cord.

BRAIN STEM AND SPINAL CORD

Caudal to the thalamus is the *brain stem*. Sometimes referred to simply as *the bulb*, the brain stem is the meeting point for neural impulses as they propagate among the cerebrum and cerebellum and the rest of the body. Many distinct groups of specialized neuron cell bodies, called nuclei, are located in the brain stem. These play roles similar to those of the subcortical nuclei in the cerebrum and cerebellum. All neural impulses pass through the brain stem on the way to and from the rest of the body.

The brain stem is almost indistinguishable from the spinal cord at its upper levels. In fact, some brain stem nuclei are located, at least in part, in the cervical segments of the spinal cord. The usual designation of tissue as being part of either the spinal cord or brain stem is simply the level of the foramen magnum.

The spinal cord is contained in the spinal canal of the spinal column, and extends in a caudal direction to the level of the intervertebral disc between the L1 and L2 vertebrae. Due to the relatively early completion of central nervous system growth when compared to skeletal growth, the spinal cord almost completely fills the spinal canal of an infant. Differential growth of the lumbar vertebrae, however, causes the spinal column to pull away inferiorly from the spinal cord at the lower levels.

The spinal cord is composed, generally, of an outer layer of whitish myelinated nerve fibers and an inner core of gray matter nuclei. The outer fibers are the major ascending and descending nerve tracts, carrying action potentials to and from the centers of the brain. The neurons of the inner core process information on the reflexive or segmental level. Such processing is done without much interaction from the higher levels of the brain, and the conscious mind is seldom aware of these functions until split seconds after they occur. Sometimes, though, the brain intervenes to consciously inhibit or coordinate reflexive spinal cord functions.

THE PERIPHERAL NERVOUS SYSTEM

The central nervous system transmits information to and receives information from the internal and external body through a series of neurons that comprise the peripheral nervous system. An individual is most often not conscious of peripheral nervous system functions until something goes wrong.

The peripheral nervous system consists of the cranial nerves, the spinal nerves, and the autonomic nervous system. We will focus on the cranial nerves and spinal nerves, since autonomic nervous functions are not usually conscious or voluntary. These include, for example, the input of blood oxygen levels and the output of smooth digestive muscle contractions. While cranial nerves and spinal nerves convey nervous impulses that are neither conscious nor voluntary, as well, they also allow muscles to contract voluntarily and deliver conscious sensory information to the central nervous system. Most speech being conscious and voluntary, it is here we will devote our attention.

CRANIAL NERVES AND SPINAL NERVES

The ultimate connection of the brain and spinal cord with the muscles of the speech mechanism is via the cranial nerves and spinal nerves. Without this connection, no sensory information would project from the end organs of sight, hearing, or touch to the conscious mind, and no muscles could operate voluntarily.

Twelve pairs of cranial nerves provide afferent and efferent communication among structures of the head and neck, including sensory areas of the skull, face, and oral cavities, as well as muscles of the face, mouth, and pharynx. These nerves have their cell bodies in the cerebrum, thalamus, and brain stem. Cell bodies for the 31 pairs of spinal nerves are located along the length of the spinal cord. Afferent spinal nerves have their cell bodies in dorsal root ganglia, just outside the spinal cord, while efferent spinal nerve branches have their cell bodies inside the cord, in the ventral horns gray.

Once the muscles contract and move the speech mechanism, an acoustic wave is created. In the listener, the acoustic wave is amplified by external and middle ear structures, and then transmitted to the inner ear. The inner ear creates nervous system impulses corresponding in many characteristics to the parameters of the acoustic wave. These begin at the inner ear, in a structure called the *cochlea*. This is where tiny cells with cilia on their free ends react to variations in fluid pressure coincident with sound energy being delivered to the middle ear by generating corresponding electrochemical changes in the eighth cranial nerve. The changes are called action potentials, and they are conveyed to successively more complex centers of the nervous system, where they are finally perceived and integrated into the listener's total psychological, cognitive, and linguistic experiences.

REFERENCES

Bak, T. H., O'Donnan, D. G., Xuereb, J. H., Boniface, S., & Hodges, J. R. (2001). Selective impairment of verb processing associated with pathological changes in Brodmann areas 44 and 45 in the motor neurone disease-dementia-aphasia syndrome. *Brain, 124,* 103-120.

Connaughton, V. M., Amiruddin, A., Clunies-Ross, K. L., French, N., & Fox A. M. (2017). Assessing hemispheric specialization for processing arithmetic skills in adults: A functional transcranial doppler ultrasonography (fTCD) study. *Journal of Neuroscience Methods, 283,* 33-41. http://dx.doi.org/10.1016/j.jneumeth.2017.03.010

Garey, L. L. (1999). *Brodmann's 'localisation in the cerebral cortex'.* London: Imperial.

Karbe, H. L., Würker, M., Herholz, K., Ghaemi, M., Pietrzyk, U., Kessler, J., & Heiss, W. D. (1995). Planum temporale and Brodmann's area 22: Magnetic resonance imaging and high-resolution positron emission tomography demonstrate functional left-right asymmetry. *Archives of Neurology, 52,* 869-74.

Nowell, M., Vos, S. B., Sidhu, M., Wilcoxen, K., Sargsyan, N., Ourselin, S., & Duncan, J. S. (2016). Meyer's loop asymmetry and language lateralisation in epilepsy. *Journal of Neurology, Neurosurgery, and Psychiatry, 87*(8), 836-842. http://doi.org/10.1136/jnnp-2015-311161

Ojemann, G., & Mateer, C. (1979). Human language cortex: Localization of memory, syntax, and sequential motor-phoneme identification systems. *Science, 205,* 1401-1403.

Penfield, W., & Boldrey, E. (1937). Somatic motor and sensory representation in the cerebral cortex of man as studied by electrical stimulation. *Brain, 60,* 389-443. https://doi.org/10.1093/brain/60.4.389

Seghier, M. L. (2013). The angular gyrus: Multiple functions and multiple subdivisions. *The Neuroscientist, 19,* 43-61. doi: 10.1177/1073858412440596

Sreedharan, R. M., Menon, A.C., James, J. S. et al. (2015). *Neuroradiology* 57: 291. doi:10.1007/s00234-014-1469-1

Wada, J. A. (1997). Youthful season revisited. *Brain and Cognition 33,* 7-10.

Zemlin, W. (1998). *Speech and hearing science: Anatomy and physiology* (4th. Ed.). Englewood Cliffs, NJ: Prentice Hall.

Part 3: Motor Functions of the Central Nervous System

GOAL

Present the general neurological organization of motor functions.

OBJECTIVES

○ Distinguish between the voluntary and involuntary motor control systems of the human nervous system.
○ Identify the specific muscular systems involved in respiration, phonation, and speech articulation.

● ● ● ● ● ● ●

MOTOR SPEECH FUNCTIONS

The role of movement in speech is so essential that even on a basic level we need a special section to cover it. Many who begin their study of the matter begin with the assumption that there is a unified brain area that triggers the contractions of speech muscles when the speaker thinks, "Go." This concept is a great oversimplification of the real motor system.

Perhaps the simplest way to consider our body's motor functions is to split them into two divisions: a *direct* or *voluntary division*, and an *indirect* or *involuntary system motor system*. Many people who are studying motor functions for the first time are surprised to discover that there is an involuntary motor system, until they consider the fact that their hearts are beating regularly and their breathing is regular without their conscious interventions. A little more contemplation leads to the conclusion that we contract a lot more muscles involuntarily than we do voluntarily.

Another factor we must consider in studying motor functions is that there are three types of muscles: *striated* or *skeletal muscles*, *smooth muscles*, and *cardiac muscles*. Muscles of each of these types function on a different basis. Striated, or skeletal, muscles are found in the head, neck, trunk, and extremities. Smooth muscles are found in the internal organs, including the digestive and respiratory tracts, and cardiac muscle is found only in the heart. Striated muscles are most susceptible to contracting under voluntary control, although they can and frequently do contract involuntarily. Both smooth and cardiac muscles contract almost entirely in an unconscious and involuntary basis.

Of the three muscle types, we will devote our attention entirely to striated or skeletal muscles, since they mediate movements of the vocal tract. Still, the fact remains that we contract and relax striated muscles more often involuntarily and unconsciously than we do voluntarily and consciously.

All skeletal or striated muscles receive the ability to contract by virtue of their connections to the central nervous system. In return, these muscles send information back to the central nervous system regarding their contractile and stretch status, their coordination with other muscles, and whether they are moving or at rest. Skeletal muscles transmit and receive their nervous system impulses via the spinal and cranial peripheral nerves, and their ability to mediate smooth, accurate, and strong movements depends largely on the quality of nerve impulses propagated via these peripheral nerves.

The cranial and spinal nerves of the peripheral nervous system contain both motor and sensory fibers. Simply put, motor fibers convey action potentials to the muscles to stimulate degrees of muscle contractions, and sensory fibers convey action potentials back to the central nervous system to ensure proper regulation of movement. Peripheral nerve motor fibers are often called the *final common pathway*, because they convey combined motor action potentials from several central nervous system nuclear pools, including the cerebral cortex, the cerebellum, basal nuclei, diverse brain stem pools, and nuclear pools in the spinal cord, all focused into the peripheral nerve.

Motor fibers of the peripheral nerves are called *lower motor neurons* and sensory fibers are called *first order sensory neurons*. If peripheral nerves are damaged or destroyed by injury or disease, the result is a deficient connection or, in the worst case, complete disconnection of the muscle from the central nervous system.

Thus, the central nervous system is unable to stimulate contraction of any kind, and the central nervous system is unaware of the contractile status of the affected muscles. Clinically, the muscle will lose tone, becoming flaccid, and wither away.

In the cerebral cortex, the gyrus at the posterior end of the frontal lobe and just in front of the central sulcus is called the precentral gyrus. In this part of the brain are located millions of cell bodies of the upper motor neurons. Upper motor neurons act in concerted response with the conscious areas of the cerebral cortex to initiate voluntary, intentional muscle contractions. From their somatotopic locations in the precentral gyrus, upper motor neurons project axons deep through the cerebral cortex, forming the corticobulbar and corticospinal tracts, known collectively as the pyramidal tracts. Axons of these tracts crossing to the contralateral side at either the caudal brain stem or the proper spinal cord segment level, to connect with the lower motor neurons, allow an individual to contract or relax skeletal muscles of the trunk and extremities volitionally.

Before any intentional movement is executed, it must be planned and programmed by the interaction of multiple cerebral cortex centers. Because these centers must work together, they are often called *association centers*. If the movements are speech movements, these centers bring many aspects of association, including memories of images formed by previous experiences, to influence multiple aspects of each speech segment. This includes stored images of the sensations associated with formations of each syllable, word and phrase. Much of this pre-programming appears to be enabled through input from and output to diverse areas of the cerebral cortex, depending upon the specific speech segments required.

It comes as a surprise to most beginning students of neurology that very few of our muscle contractions and relaxations are intentional. This is probably because we are only conscious of our intentional movements until something goes awry with the unconscious ones. Motor tracts that react to intentional input from the voluntary motor system and maintain muscle tonus and skeletal posture over various body inclinations are called *extrapyramidal tracts*. These tracts ensure smooth, accurate movement and appropriate initiations and cessations of movements.

One example of unconscious muscle contractions is found in the relatively effortless way we reciprocally contract and relax opposing muscles. For example, when we wish to lift a coffee cup from a table, we will contract the biceps (brachii) while simultaneously, and at the same rate, relaxing the opposing triceps (brachii).

Such synergistic contraction and relaxation are performed smoothly and unconsciously through passive processing by motor nuclei in the cerebellum. The cerebellum responds, in part, to input from the motor cerebral cortex and sensory feedback from the muscles. In the vocal tract, reciprocal muscle contractions enable precise elevation of the tongue apex through contraction of the tongue's superior longitudinal muscle and simultaneous relaxation of the inferior longitudinal muscle. Tongue protrusion and retraction would be troublesome without synergistic functioning of the genioglossus, palatoglossus, and styloglossus muscles.

Cerebellar input is facilitated by input from special collections of neuron cell bodies deep in the cerebral hemispheres and in the brain stem. These collections of neuron cell bodies are called the *basal nuclei and associated structures*. Together they form a loop of neural regulation that facilitates the smooth, accurate and controlled execution of complex muscle contractions. Subcortical centers respond to input from the motor tracts as they pass through the deep areas of the cerebral hemispheres on their way to the brain stem. Other input comes from the thalamus, the cerebellum, and neighboring nuclear centers, to ensure smooth, accurate, and controlled movement, even when movements are unconscious. Basal nuclei and associated structures react to this input by projecting neural output to the thalamus, cerebral cortex, brain stem nuclei, and cerebellum (Bostana, Duma, & Strick, 2010).

MUSCLES OF SPEECH AND THE NERVOUS SYSTEM

Any discussion of motor speech functions is incomplete without including the muscles. The muscles of speech are the motor end-organs that respond to output from the central nervous system and send sensory feedback to the central nervous system. Voluntary, conscious output from the central nervous system is conveyed via lower motor neurons, and sensory feedback is conveyed via first order sensory neurons, all of which are grouped in spinal and cranial nerves. In turn, muscular contractions move the peripheral speech mechanism, affecting changes in air pressure and creating the sounds, or phones, that form the raw signals by which we attribute meaning to the spoken signal. These air pressure changes are propagated to the peripheral hearing mechanisms of the listener.

Speech muscles can be generally grouped into five broad categories: *respiratory muscles, phonatory muscles, oral muscles, velopharyngeal muscles,* and *facial muscles*. All these groups work in concert.

RESPIRATORY MUSCLES

Respiratory muscles are often grouped into inspiratory and expiratory categories, depending upon whether their contractions bring air into the respiratory system or force air out. Their contractions are most often involuntary and generally unconscious, being functions of the autonomic branch of the peripheral nervous system. For speaking purposes, however, contractions of respiratory muscles are voluntary and conscious.

Thus, muscles of inspiration bring air into the respiratory system, and muscles of expiration force air out. They do this by respectively increasing and decreasing thoracic volume. When muscles of inspiration contract, the diaphragm flattens and expands the chest cavity in a superior-inferior dimension, while the intercostal muscles act on the rib cage to pull the first six ribs forward and upward, and the seventh through tenth ribs laterally, increasing volume in those dimensions. As the chest wall expands, the lungs and alveoli follow suit. Increased volume decreases internal air pressure and draws air into the system. Relaxing the inspiratory muscles reverses the process, compressing the chest, lungs, and alveoli; increasing internal air pressure; and forcing respiratory gases out.

In normal function, at least for egressive speech sounds—that is, speech sounds created by the power of air leaving the vocal tract—muscles of inspiration are most active. This fact seems ironic to some since inspiratory muscle contractions increase the volume of the lungs and draw air into the system, and most speech is accomplished by the power of air leaving the system. However, unless for some special circumstance a speaker desires to forcefully expel air from the lungs, say, for shouting or trying to squeeze every last syllable per milliliter of air out of the lungs, the usual function is to slowly let air out of the system in order to use the volume of air for the longest period. This means slowly relaxing the tonic state of inspiratory muscles until the normal thoracic relaxation state is reached, then re-inflating at a convenient pause to continue speaking. Note that the respiratory muscles function automatically during breathing and voluntarily during speech.

The main inspiratory muscles are the diaphragm and 11 pairs of external and internal intercostal muscles. Contraction of the diaphragm flattens the muscle and increases superior-inferior dimension of the thorax. Intercostal muscle contractions are more complex and bring about expansion or contraction of the thorax depending upon their locations along the thoracic wall (De Troyer, Kirkwood, & Wilson, 2005). External intercostal muscles bring about thoracic expansion if they are located in the rostral and dorsal regions of the rib cage, gradually reversing their roles to chest compressors in the caudal and ventral regions. Internal intercostal muscles cause the chest to expand if they are located in the rostral and ventral rib cage, giving way to thoracic compression as their location progresses to caudal and dorsal segments. The direction of thoracic expansion is anterior and superior (pump handle movement) as well as lateral (bucket handle movement). These provide adequate thoracic expansion for most purposes, including normal speaking and tidal breathing.

If a speaker desires to achieve the maximum thoracic expansion, drawing in that ultimate small volume of air, the secondary or accessory muscles of inspiration are brought into play to supplement the primary muscles. Such a need might arise if a speaker intended to impose the absolute maximum number of syllables on a full breath, or if a singer wanted to hold a note for the longest duration possible. Secondary muscles might also be helpful if a speaker had a pathological condition that limited the amount of air accessible for speaking. These muscles expand the chest wall by moving ribs and shoulders anteriorly, superiorly, and laterally.

Muscles of expiration may also be recruited for speaking under circumstances that demand the greatest volume of air as a power source, or occasionally if a great increase in sound pressure is desired for activities such as cheering on the home team or some other highly unusual vocal activity. Muscles of expiration oppose those of inspiration and are brought into play according to demand. Thus, muscles that oppose diaphragmatic contraction are those abdominal muscles that push abdominal contents up against the flattened diaphragm. Those that oppose muscles of thoracic expansion are ones that compress the chest.

Primary and secondary respiratory muscles connect to the central nervous system via sensory and motor branches of spinal nerves projecting from cervical through lumbar spinal cord segments. Multiple central nervous system tracts control and regulate voluntary and automatic contractions. Whether or not respiratory muscle contractions are voluntary, the same lower motor neurons stimulate their contractions. The lower motor neurons that connect the diaphragm to the central nervous system are motor branches of cervical spinal nerves C3, C4, and C5, combined to form the phrenic nerve. The intercostal muscles receive their lower motor innervation from the motor branches of the thoracic spinal nerves, T1 through T11.

Other muscles of the head and neck resist the egress of air during the act of speaking. The tonic status of these muscles adjusts in concert with the relaxation of thoracic expanders. Facial muscles, particularly those that control the oral opening, function during the articulation of labial consonants, rounded vowels, and some idiolectic variations of alveolar and postalveolar fricatives. Within the oral cavity, lingual muscles impede airflow to varying extents, ranging from complete blockage during plosive articulation to mild resistance during mid-open vowel and articulation of /r/ and /j/. Cervical muscles also impede the flow of air during speech, especially the glottal adductors and vocal ligament tensors during phonation.

Facial muscles receive their lower motor innervation via cranial nerve VII, also called the facial nerve. Inside the oral cavity, the hypoglossal nerve, cranial nerve XII, controls the intrinsic tongue muscles and all the extrinsic tongue muscles except the palatoglossus muscles, served by cranial nerve X, the vagus nerve. The same vagus nerve, with help from cranial nerves IX and XI (glossopharyngeal and accessory nerves) forming the pharyngeal plexus, provides for central nervous system connections with the pharyngeal musculature.

PHONATORY MUSCLES

Muscles that produce and modify the phonatory source are intrinsic to the larynx. The larynx is located in the lower pharynx, and is technically part of the respiratory system. For speech scientists, though, the muscles of the larynx are of special interest, since the vocal folds adduct for production of most phonemes. Intrinsic laryngeal muscles adduct and abduct the vocal folds to start or stop voicing, adjust tension on the vocal folds to change pitch and resist the flow of air, and adjust the area of the laryngeal inlet. While adjusting the area of the laryngeal inlet may not be of much speech use, it is extremely important in swallowing. The other two functions are, of course, essential to segmental and suprasegmental speech.

Like the muscles of the upper pharynx, the muscles of the larynx receive most of their motor innervation via the vagus nerve (cranial nerve X). This includes voluntary motor functions as well as involuntary motor functions, although some discussion about voluntary motor functions is in order. Fibers projecting from

the vagus nerve cell bodies in the brain stem combine with fibers projecting from the nucleus ambiguus as the accessory nerve (cranial nerve XI) to provide what has been classically distinguished as voluntary, in contrast to autonomic, motor innervation of the pharyngeal muscles (Tubbs, Benninger, Loukas, & Cohen-Gadol, 2014). Sensory feedback is conveyed from the pharynx to the central nervous system via the vagus nerve.

ORAL MUSCLES, VELOPHARYNGEAL MUSCLES, AND FACIAL MUSCLES

The muscles of the oral cavity, velopharynx and face can be considered as a functional group. They act in concert to modify the voiced or unvoiced airstream for speech articulation.

The oral musculature that acts in the production of phonemes is located both inside and just outside the oral cavity. Muscles inside the cavity act in the production of phonemes created by tongue and velar movements. This includes all the vowels and all but the labial consonants. Speech-related muscles located outside the oral cavity are grouped as muscles of facial expression, muscles of mandibular elevation, and muscles of the larynx.

Intraoral muscles include the intrinsic and extrinsic tongue muscles and the muscles of the velopharyngeal sphincter. Intrinsic lingual muscles have their origins and insertions within the body of the tongue, and their contractions change the shape of the tongue within the oral cavity. Such movements include the elevation of the tongue apex for alveolar and dental articulation and the raising of the tongue's blade for palatal articulation. Extrinsic tongue muscles insert in the tongue's body, but originate elsewhere. Extrinsic muscles change the position of the tongue within the oral cavity, moving it forward and backward, up and down for dental, palatal, velar uvular, and even pharyngeal consonant articulations, as well as front, central, and back; and open and close vowel articulations.

Muscles of the velopharynx elevate the velum to separate the oropharynx and oral cavity from the nasopharynx and nasal cavity. When the velum is lowered, ether actively or passively, the nasopharynx and nasal cavity become parts of the resonating vocal tract system. Outside the oral cavity, the facial muscles and the laryngeal muscles are employed in speaking, and the muscles of mandibular elevation keep the tongue and lips in useful proximity to fixed speech structures in the upper oral cavity and pharynx. Muscles of facial expression play their roles in speech articulation by contracting to either round or spread the lips, bring the lips into contact with each other, and bring the lower lip into contact with the upper teeth. These movements are essential to the articulation of labial consonants and lip rounding-spreading.

Other muscles outside the oral cavity elevate or depress the mandible. These muscles also play important roles in mastication. For speech purposes, mandibular elevation is required for all but the most open vowels, and the velar and glottal consonants. Mandibular depression is not required for most speech, but is desirable in cases where the greatest acoustic amplitude is important. While the speech purposes of the laryngeal muscles are most often considered as producing the voice (phonatory source), they also play a role in consonant articulation. The glottal plosive, /ʔ/, and two glottal fricatives, /ɦ/ and /h/, are produced by articulation of the opposing vocal folds.

Nervous system functions of the articulatory muscles are both sensory and motor, and they can be contracted consciously and unconsciously, and voluntarily and involuntarily. Speech movements are, for the most part, voluntary (Simmonds, Leech, Collins, Redjep, & Wise, 2014). Most treatment of the articulatory system focuses on the rapid and variable feats of motor action, but none would be accurate or coordinated without sensory feedback to the central nervous system.

Lower motor neurons that connect the intraoral musculature with the central nervous system for voluntary and involuntary contractions include the hypoglossal nerve for the intrinsic and extrinsic tongue muscles, the vagus-accessory (forming, with the glossopharyngeal nerve, the pharyngeal plexus) and trigeminal nerves for the velopharyngeal sphincter, and the trigeminal nerve for mandibular elevation. Sensory output to the central nervous system is accomplished via the trigeminal nerve and the glossopharyngeal nerve on both sides.

Facial muscles contract via stimuli delivered through the facial nerve, and glottal muscles contract by means of action motor action potentials delivered via the vagus-accessory nerve complex. Sensation from the face and anterior two-thirds of the oral cavity is conveyed via the trigeminal nerve, while sensation from the posterior one-third of the oral cavity is conveyed via the glossopharyngeal and vagus nerves. Interestingly, the muscles of facial expression quite often contract involuntarily, in response to emotional states, and such emotional contractions can interfere with speech articulation.

REFERENCES

Bostana, A. C., Duma, R. P., & Strick, P. L. (2010). The basal ganglia communicate with the cerebellum. *Proceedings of the National Academy of Sciences of the United States of America, 107,* 8452-8456. doi: 10.1073/pnas.1000496107

De Troyer, A, Kirkwood P. A., & Wilson, T. A. (2005). Respiratory action of the intercostal muscles. *Physiology Review, 85,* 717-756.

Simmonds, A. J., Leech, R., Collins, C., Redjep, O., & Wise, R. J. S. (2014). Sensory-motor integration during speech production localizes to both left and right plana temporale. *The Journal of Neuroscience, 34,* 12963-12972. http://doi.org/10.1523/JNEUROSCI.0336-14.2014

Tubbs, R. S., Benninger, B., Loukas, M., & Cohen-Gadol, A. A. (2014). Cranial roots of the accessory nerve exist in the majority of adult humans. *Clinical Anatomy, 27,* 102-107. doi:10.1002/ca.22125

Part 4: Listening

GOAL

Examine the neurological basis for speech perception.

OBJECTIVES

- Recognize the extent and functions of the peripheral hearing system.
- Recognize the extent and functions of the central hearing system.
- Identify two hearing functions of cranial nerve VIII.
- Distinguish among the four levels of auditory processing.
- Trace central auditory pathways from the cochlear nuclei to the cerebral cortical centers.

• • • • • • •

STAGES OF LISTENING

Since the main purpose of speaking is to convey information, a listener is required. This is true even if one is speaking to oneself. In fact, one might argue that the listener is most often the speaker, since monitoring one's own spoken output, and correcting it when necessary, is a good way to ensure the message is conveyed.

We will discuss self-monitoring presently. First, though, we will treat the topic of listening by others who are interested in what the speaker has to say.

Speech reception and subsequent central processing can be described in a simplified way as consisting of four stages (Porch, 1981): *reception, perception, association,* and *integration.* For these purposes, we define reception as the conversion of speech acoustics into neural impulses and their propagation to the auditory receptive centers in the brain stem and cerebral cortex, perception as the recognition of differences in the speech signal, association as the linguistic processing of the perceived signal into meaningful content, and integration as the personality processes involved in dealing with the information.

During speech reception, physical signals are converted into neural action potentials. Physiologically, reception is accomplished through combined peripheral and central functions. The external and middle ears gather and amplify the spoken signal, and the inner ear brain stem auditory pathways begin sorting the signal for subsequent processing. Efficient transmission of a spoken signal depends on the functions of these receptive structures. Any anomalies in either peripheral or central auditory functions compromise subsequent central processing.

The second level is perception. Here, the brain sorts and differentiates the basic characteristics of the neural potentials. Special processes at the perceptual level include discrimination, the ability to distinguish small differences among similar signals. A special kind of discrimination is figure-ground discrimination, the ability to distinguish a signal against competing background noise. Two other important perceptual processes are *closure,* the process of inferring a complete signal after a partial presentation, and *sequencing,* the ability to recognize temporal contiguity of events.

Association relates the listener's perceptions to whatever meanings or symbolic referent functions are stored in the memory. A listener's associations may or may not be the same as those of a speaker. Herein lies a much-discussed problem inherent in human communication.

Integration of spoken communication in the listener's mind combines presently processed signals with previously processed information. When novel associations arrive, they can be stored for subsequent interactions. At this stage, a listener may decide to respond or not. Interestingly, association might also be considered a part of output, since the differences are blurred at this point.

Figure 5.4-1. Anatomists often divide the ear into three main sections. (SVETLANA VERBINSKAYA/ Shutterstock.com)

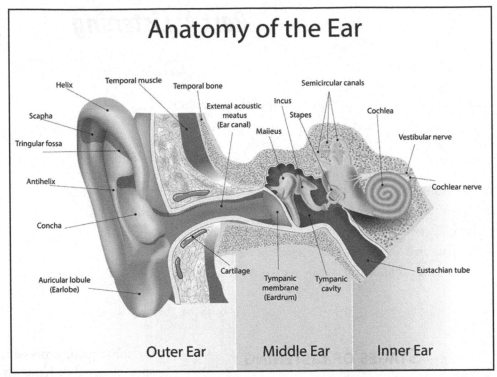

Anatomy of the Ear

Helix
Temporal muscle
Temporal bone
Scapha
External acoustic meatus (Ear canal)
Tringular fossa
Semicircular canals
Incus
Stapes
Maiieus
Cochlea
Vestibular nerve
Antihelix
Cochlear nerve
Concha
Cartilage
Eustachian tube
Auricular lobule (Earlobe)
Tympanic membrane (Eardrum)
Tympanic cavity

Outer Ear   Middle Ear   Inner Ear

REVIEW OF THE PERIPHERAL AUDITORY SYSTEM

It should be apparent that the best central associations depend upon the most accurate transformations of the spoken acoustic signal to neural impulses. This is a function of the peripheral hearing mechanism, consisting of the external, middle, and inner ear. First of all, we will have a brief review of the anatomy of the hearing system. (For more detail, consult your anatomy or audiology text.)

As you may recall, the hearing system may be studied in two main divisions: a peripheral hearing system, and a central hearing system. The peripheral hearing system begins at the pinna, the visible part of the ear, and extends to the cranial nerve VIII, also known as the vestibulocochlear nerve, synapses in the brain stem at one of two cochlear nuclei on each side (see Figure 5.4-1).

The peripheral hearing system has three functions: to selectively amplify acoustic energy from the environment, to aid in localization of a sound source, and to transform acoustic energy into neurochemical potentials. Outer and middle ear structures selectively amplify acoustic energy. Transduction of mechanical energy into neurochemical energy occurs in the hair cells of the basilar membrane. Interestingly, these cells

are differentially sensitive to certain frequencies, and are arranged along the basilar membrane with sensitivity to higher frequencies at the basal end and to lower frequencies at the apical end. This arrangement is called *tonotopic.*

Neural impulses generated in concert with the mechanical (acoustic) energy at the basilar membrane are conveyed along axons of the spiral ganglion in either inner ear. In the nervous system, a *ganglion* is generally defined as a collection of neuron cell bodies in the peripheral nervous system. This ganglion is named the spiral ganglion because it winds around the 2¾ turns of the cochlea. Nerve fibers (axons) projecting from these cell bodies aggregate into one of two divisions of the eighth cranial nerve, also known as the vestibulocochlear nerve. Cranial nerve VIII has two main divisions: a vestibular division, which conveys action potentials associated with head position to the central nervous system, and a cochlear division, which conveys action potentials associated with sound to the central nervous system.

The cochlear division of VIII, in turn, has two divisions: one for transmission of acoustic information to be discriminated, and another for conveying non-discriminatory, reflex impulses. The reflex division is part of the survival mechanism and not usually associated with speech, so we will focus on the discriminatory division.

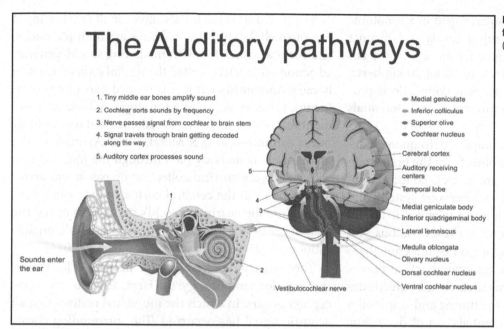

Figure 5.4-2. Auditory pathways, from external ear to cerebral cortex. (Studio BKK/Shutterstock.com)

The discriminatory division of the vestibulocochlear nerve enables the listener to discriminate among acoustic frequencies between 20 Hertz and 20 kilohertz. Perception of speech depends upon the ability to discriminate among complex sounds, and the sounds of speech are well within these frequency parameters. Analysis and perception depend upon psychological factors, and such factors are also neurological functions. Sensory fibers VIII destined for the discriminatory pathways connect with single higher-level neurons for greater discrimination. Most of the higher-level discriminatory terminations are situated in the ventral cochlear nucleus, while axons conveying reflexively initiated auditory impulses terminate at the dorsal cochlear nuclei. Both tracts make connections with neuron cell bodies in the central auditory system at these cochlear nuclei.

A nucleus is a collection of neuron cell bodies in the central nervous system, just as a ganglion is a collection of cell bodies in the peripheral nervous system. The ventral and dorsal cochlear nuclei are located roughly in the middle of the brain stem, and mark the division between the central auditory system and the peripheral auditory system. There are several nuclei in the central auditory tracts, and they are important landmarks of diagnostic significance.

REVIEW OF THE CENTRAL AUDITORY SYSTEM

The central auditory system consists of neural pathways from the brain stem to the cerebral cortex, as well as neurons of the cortex, itself. It begins at the cochlear nuclei and extends to the cerebral cortex.

FUNCTION OF THE CENTRAL AUDITORY SYSTEM

The function of the central auditory system is to further refine the processing of auditory impulses originating in the peripheral system. Such neural impulses, originating in the periphery and conveyed to the central nervous system, are called *afferent impulses*.

THE CENTRAL AUDITORY PATHWAYS

As we said earlier, the central division of the auditory system begins at synapses of the vestibulocochlear nerve (VIII) fibers with the cell bodies in the cochlear nuclei of the brain stem. These cell bodies, two of which are located on each side of the brain stem in an area called the *pons,* are the beginning of the central pathways (see Figure 5.4-2).

The vestibulocochlear nerve bifurcates, or divides in two, in this location, sending fibers to one or the other of the two cochlear nuclei. One branch goes to the dorsal cochlear nucleus for reflexive hearing. Another branch goes to the ventral cochlear nucleus for discriminatory hearing.

The cochlear nuclei are also arranged in a tonotopic pattern. That is, they have subdivisions and distinct regions associated with acoustic frequency, in the audible range from about 20 Hertz to about 20 kilohertz. Within the cochlear nuclei, neuron connections provide many combinations to process action potentials generated by acoustic input.

The central auditory pathways are frequently described in terms of synaptic points from the brain stem to the cortex. These points are nuclei, collections of neuron cell bodies in the central nervous system, and nerve fiber projections from the various cell bodies have connections called *synapses* at these locations. Not all axons connect at the synaptic points, but enough do that the progress of a sound generated action potential can be traced from nucleus to nucleus by electrodes placed on the skull's surface. The timing and amplitudes of these sound-generated potentials are of diagnostic significance to hearing specialists.

The first synapse in the auditory pathway is the superior olivary complex. It is located in the middle part of the brain stem, in the pons, a little rostral to the cochlear nuclei. Each superior olive receives fibers from the (anterior) VCN. At this point, about 85% of nerve fibers originating in the cochlear nuclei cross, or decussate, from one side to the other side. This means that acoustic impulses received in one ear are processed on the opposite side of the central nervous system.

Other central auditory nerve fibers, some of which synapse at the superior olive and some of which that do not, course rostrally along the brain stem from the pons to the midbrain. Olivocochlear bundle fibers propagate back to the cochlea and convey otoacoustic emissions, which are of diagnostic significance to hearing specialists.

Fibers emanating from the superior olivary complex form a flat collection of axons called a *lemniscus*. (Lemniscus means "ribbon" in Greek, and the axons which form this ribbon course rostrally.) This one is called the *lateral lemniscus*. There is a synapse in the lateral lemniscus, called, appropriately enough, the *nucleus of the lateral lemniscus*.

The next synapse is the inferior colliculus, located in the part of the brain stem known as the midbrain. The midbrain is at the rostral end of the brain stem. Not all fibers synapse here, either, but all collect and course rostrally. The inferior colliculi are notable as centers for non-discriminatory hearing. Here are found visual and somatic connections with auditory fibers.

The thalamus is the relay center for all sensory input except smell. Within the thalamus are multiple nuclei, and the one associated with mediating sound-generated action potentials is called the *medial geniculate body*, because anatomists felt it was shaped like a knee joint (genu). Here, evidence of a tonotopic cellular arrangement that was observed in the cochlea and the cochlear nuclei continues (Imig & Morel, 1985). Axons from the medial geniculate body pass through the internal capsule, a deep, subcortical collection of axons, and arrive at cell bodies in the cerebral cortex, at the primary receptive site for hearing, Heschl's gyrus, also called the *auditory cortex*. There is evidence of tonotopic organization here, as well (Leaver & Rauschecker, 2016).

The primary receptive site for hearing is located in the superior temporal gyrus. Here, the process of reception occurs, in which the individual realizes that an acoustic signal has occurred. The surrounding cortex is the auditory association cortex in which perceptive associative and integrative functions, described earlier in this section, are processed. Each hemisphere receives input from each ear.

PROCESSING OF SPEECH

Processing of speech is, of course, very complex. Earlier, we noted that it takes place on at least four levels. Yet all speech processing may not be done on a purely receptive level. There is a large body of evidence to suggest that we process speech in terms of how we, ourselves, speak, bringing in to play the expressive components of speech processing as part of the receptive functions (e.g., Casserly & Pisoni, 2010).

In considering speech or, more accurately, spoken language processing, then, many refer to anterior versus posterior centers. Anterior centers are more associative for motor output, and linguistic symbolic decoding and encoding is felt to be posterior, but it is clear that both have expressive and receptive functions. It is also apparent that much more widespread speech processing occurs in cortical and subcortical brain areas. Associative cortical centers are progressively removed from the primary receptive sites, and may be considered meeting points for various kinds of signal processing by other parts of the brain. In addition to cortical centers, subcortical structures, including the thalamus, have roles in speech processing. These roles have yet to be fully explored.

REFERENCES

Casserly, E. D., & Pisoni, D. B. (2010). Speech perception and production. *Wiley Interdisciplinary Reviews. Cognitive Science, 1,* 629–647. http://doi.org/10.1002/wcs.63

Imig, T. J., & Morel, A. (1985). Tonotopic organization in ventral nucleus of medial geniculate body in the cat. *Journal of Neurophysiology, 53,* 309-340.

Leaver, A. M., & Rauschecker, J. P. (2016). Functional topography of human auditory cortex. *Journal of Neuroscience, 36,* 1416-1428.

Porch, B. E. (1981). *Porch index of communicative ability: Volume 2, third edition, administration, scoring and interpretation.* Palo Alto, CA: Consulting Psychologists Press.

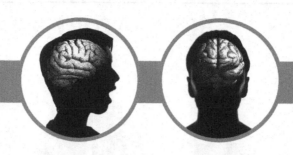

Speech Systems

This chapter covers the basics of the functional roles of three subsystems of speech: *respiration*, *phonation*, and *articulation*. All three subsystems function as a concerted unity to produce the wonderfully varied manners of speaking. With seemingly little or no effort, we quickly inflate our lungs and let the air out in concert with the interplay of our vocal tract musculature. Since the majority of speech begins with an outward flow of air from the lungs to the mouth and nose, we will begin with the respiratory power source and move distally to the contributions of the laryngeal, oral, and nasal cavities.

Part 1: Respiration and Speech

GOAL

Examine the role of the respiratory system in speech.

OBJECTIVES

○ Recognize the role of the respiratory system in speech.
○ Distinguish among the nomenclature and average values of four respiratory capacities:
  ▪ Vital Capacity
  ▪ Tidal Volume
  ▪ Inspiratory Reserve
  ▪ Expiratory Reserve
○ Distinguish speech breathing from tidal breathing.
○ Distinguish muscular forces from relaxation forces in respiration.
○ Distinguish among alveolar pressure, relaxation pressure, and abdominal pressure.

Culbertson, W. R.
Fundamentals of the Speech and Language Sciences (pp 79-106).
© 2020 Taylor & Francis Group.

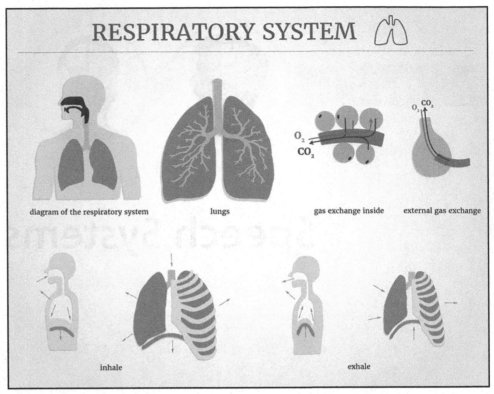

The role of the respiratory system in speech is to create pressurized air flow (see Figure 6.1-1). It is often said that the respiratory system provides the power for speech, and in this case, the power is *pneumatic* power.

For most speaking purposes, air flows from the lungs outward to the lips and nares. Speech sounds produced in this manner are termed *egressive*, made by the pressure of air leaving the respiratory system. The flow of air drives the displacement of structures such as the vocal folds and, less noticeably, oral structures during running speech. It creates pressure differentials across vocal tract constrictions to enable a speaker to articulate plosives and fricatives. Airflow modifications also contribute to changes in loudness and pitch.

In physical terms, the kinetic energy of pressurized pulmonary air is modified to create acoustic sources. You will recall that pressure is a quantity derived by dividing force by the surface over which it is applied. In this case, the force is the energy of compressed air, and the surfaces over which the force is applied are the outer layers of the vocal tract structures, particularly the vocal folds. In order to create speech, air pressure must perform work on vocal tract structures. Work is a quantity derived by multiplying force applied over a distance, and energy is the capacity to do work. For speech, energy is created by the pressure of compressed air in the respiratory system. That energy is expressed as sound (a form of mechanical energy) and heat (thermodynamic energy) to create pressure differentials.

Most languages use egressive airflow to produce phonemes. When air flows from the distal parts of the vocal tract into the proximal parts of the respiratory system, the flow is called *ingressive*. Ingressive airflow is occasional in most languages, but as paralinguistic phenomena, such as gasps or snorts. In some languages, ingressive speech is a normal phonetic feature (Eklund, 2008).

The essential role of the respiratory system in speech is overlooked by some in favor of the more obvious articulatory or phonatory functions, but without the respiratory system as a pneumatic driving force, vocal communication is very difficult. In fact, a large part of the field of communication sciences and disorders is devoted to studying the effects and treatment of individuals for whom the respiratory system is compromised or even disconnected from the phonatory and articulatory mechanisms as the result of congenital anomaly, disease, injury, or surgery.

Speech sounds created with egressive air flowing from or to the lungs and lower respiratory tract are termed *pulmonic*. The International Phonetic Association (IPA) offers a chart on its website (https://www.internationalphoneticassociation.org/) indicating place manner and voicing characteristics of a number of pulmonic consonants, suggesting that these require air flowing from the lower respiratory tract in order to be heard.

Lacking effective support from the respiratory system, a speaker is required to use non-pulmonic sounds, created by impounding air at the place of articulation and releasing it, either egressively or ingressively. Non-pulmonic consonants include clicks, implosives, and ejectives. Individuals whose vocal tracts are disconnected from the lower respiratory system often learn to use non-pulmonic consonants as syllable boundaries, and learning to create syllables with non-pulmonic consonants is a frequent learning outcome activity in speech therapy for rehabilitation following laryngectomy.

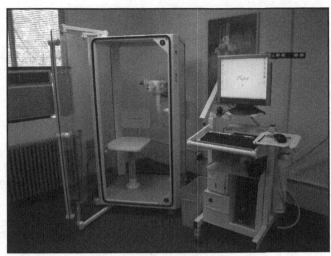

Figure 6.1-2. Spirometer. ("Body Plethysmography chamber 01.jpg" by Joe Mabel / used under CC BY-SA 3.0 / Desaturated from original)

RESPIRATORY VOLUMES

In order for the respiratory system to create pressure changes, air must be impounded and temporarily stored in the lungs and/or respiratory passages. At least part of the storage system must be variable in volume so pressure can be modified and create the conditions that make air flow from one location to another. The quantities of these variable volumes are important to the study of respiratory function in general and to the study of respiratory function in speech in particular. It will be recalled that the International System of Units (SI) derivation for volume is length³. The SI standard unit for volume (or capacity) is the liter (l), which equates to 1,000 cm³ or 1,000 cc.

Respiratory volumes can be quantified by using a *spirometer* (see Figure 6.1-2). Spirometric data are useful in monitoring the respiratory health of individuals, and they are also useful in conducting scientific research on speech. A spirometer uses a computerized or analog visual recording to show changes in an individual's respiratory volumes and air flow over time. For the study of speech, the most important of these volumes are *vital capacity, tidal volume, inspiratory reserve*, and *expiratory reserve* (see Figure 6.1-3).

Vital capacity is the total volume of air that can be expired after a maximum inspiration. It is easy to appreciate that this is the volume of air functionally available to an individual. The magnitude of vital capacity varies considerably among individuals, depending upon their size, age, gender, health status, and posture. According to Blom (2004), vital capacity is generally about 75% to 80% of total lung capacity. Backman et al. (2015) reported a range from 3.73 l, in a group of 244 adult females, to 5.45 l, in a group of 237 adult males.

Variability was wide, with standard deviations of 0.94 l and 0.81 l, respectively.

To measure vital capacity, the person to be tested is asked to inspire as deeply as possible, then to expire through a tube until no more air is available. A clinician is usually nearby to coach and encourage the individual during the process, since such efforts can be quite variable both within a patient and among patients. In extended durations of speech, inspired air is released as slowly as possible and ultimately pushed out forcefully in order to extend the duration of the utterance. If a person wished to extend an utterance or phonate a vowel for as long as possible, nearly the same maneuver required to measure vital capacity would produce the desired results, although the last few syllables would sound awkward.

Most speech, however, is produced with the intention of speaking for short durations, and normally occurs in short bursts. Conversational speech requires a quick shallow inspiration, followed by a slow expiration to produce the desired air pressures. For this kind of speech, *tidal volumes*, or the volumes used during normal respiratory cycles, are sufficient. The word tidal is used to capture the sense of a normal and constant ebb and flow of air over time, like the ocean tides. For most people, tidal volume is about 0.5 l.

On occasions when more duration is desired for longer utterances, *reserve volumes* may be used. One can inspire more air than the amount inspired during tidal breathing, and the same is true for expiration. If a speaker is aware that there is a need for a longer utterance, such as might be needed when delivering a speech, singing, or reciting a dialogue, an extra volume

Figure 6.1-3. Smoothed respiratory volumes as depicted by spirometry. (Image drawn by Mathew DeVore)

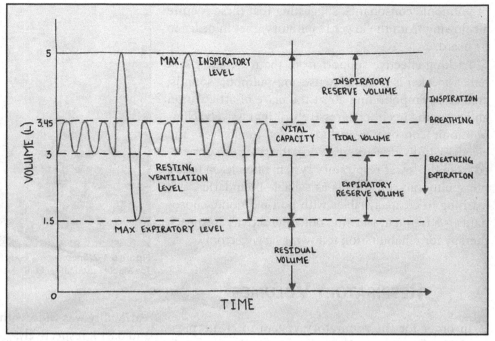

of air can be inspired beyond the normal tidal inspiration. Similarly, if the inspired volume is found to be insufficient, the speaker may continue to power the speech mechanism with air pressure produced by contracting the thorax beyond the resting state of tidal expiration. At their extremes, reserve volumes are rather not as efficient as tidal and mid-reserve volumes in providing a consistent, even power source for speech (Binazzi et al., 2006).

Inspiratory reserve, sometimes called *complemental air*, is the volume that can be inspired beyond the tidal inspiration. It represents about 50% of total lung capacity (Blom, 2004). Inspiratory reserve volumes would usually be applied in cases where a speaker anticipates an extended speech or other voicing duration, such as singing. At the peak levels of lung capacity, the recoil pressure is relatively strong, and vocal tract muscular efforts are usually too effortful to produce efficient or normal sounding speech.

Similarly, expiratory reserve volume, the volume that can be expired beyond tidal expiration, is normally accompanied by a diminishing flow rate. Expiratory reserve capacity is about 15% to 20% of total lung capacity (Blom, 2004) and would typically be used by an untrained speaker who had more to say than breath to support the effort. As airflow rate diminishes, the aerodynamics of the vocal tract become less efficient as drivers of speech sources, requiring muscular effort to predominate. Expiratory reserve volume is sometimes called *supplemental air*.

RESPIRATORY CYCLES

The flow of air in and out of the respiratory system can be described in cyclic terms. Each cycle would, thus, consist of an *inspiratory phase* and an *expiratory phase*, and one cycle would be considered one inspiration and one expiration. In this sense, the words inspiration and expiration are synonymous with the words inhalation and exhalation. The inspiratory and expiratory phases of a respiratory cycle differ in duration according to the uses to which the flow of air is put. Thus, the inspiratory phase of a tidal respiratory cycle takes a little less than half of the entire cycle, while the inspiratory phase of a respiratory cycle for a long duration utterance takes about 20% of the entire cycle.

BREATHING FOR SPEECH

In the most general terms, the difference between speech breathing and tidal breathing lies in the timing. As described above, volumes may differ depending upon speaking requirements. Timing of speech breathing may be generally described as a quick, full inspiration and a slow expiration, with inspiration taking much less time in the speech respiratory cycle than it does in the tidal cycle, and expiration taking much more time.

However, breathing for speech purposes is very much more complex than the general description above because it depends upon the needs of the speaker. The speaker consciously or unconsciously determines a rate and volume of air flow we shall refer to as the *desired flow*. Desired flow needs are far too complex to be seen as simple active inspiration and passive, steady-state expiration. Instead, different speech needs, postures, and physical conditions cause a constant variation in the way a speaker may desire air to flow in and out of the respiratory system.

Speech needs include the use of pauses and inflections, and changes in loudness or in the context of speech. These, of course, will change the desired air flow needs. If a speaker desires to shout, for instance, greater subglottic pressure and greater air flow will be required as compared to the desired air flow for a short, whispered utterance.

Postural changes also affect the way the respiratory system functions in speech. If the speaker is supine, for example, changes in the way the abdomen pushes on the thorax change the relationship of muscular effort needed to produce a desired air flow. This is an important consideration in clinical applications for patients confined to the bed.

Varying constitutional or physical conditions also affect the way the respiratory system functions in speech. States of physical exertion, for example, are easy to identify with respiratory changes needed for desired flow. Remembering that respiration is primarily used to support metabolism, the speaker who is exhausted will have very different air flow needs than one who is rested, as will one with respiratory pathology. Another consideration is environmental. If there is a lot of ambient noise, for example, one might expect to observe compensatory changes in respiratory speech function to create additional speech loudness compared with respiratory speech function in quiet conditions.

Kinetic Theory of Gases

Movement of air in and out of the respiratory system, whether for speaking or quiet breathing, depends upon principles of the *Kinetic Theory of Gases*, postulated by Daniel Bernoulli in 1738. This principle is based in part on the assumption that gases consist of molecules in constant motion. So far, that assumption has withstood much scrutiny. The molecules in a gas are in constant, random motion; they are neither attracted to nor repelled by one another, but rather bounce back and forth through space and occasionally collide. If their temperature increases, molecules have more

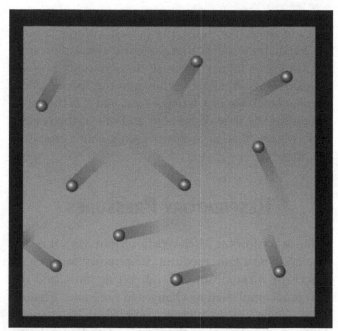

Figure 6.1-4. Random motion of gas particles creates gas pressure. ("Kinetic theory of gases.svg" by Sharayanan / used under CC BY-SA 3.0 / Desaturated from original)

energy with which to bounce around, and the greater energy translates into more pressure on the interior of any volume in which they are contained. The inverse is also true: the more bounciness they have, the hotter they get. Their motion can be concurrently described in terms of their temperature or pressure.

Equal amounts of the same gas have the same number of molecules (*molecular volume*). If equal molecular volumes of the same gas are confined in containers with different internal volumes, the molecules in the smaller volume will be squeezed closer together and, because they are in constant, random motion (see Figure 6.1-4), exerting force over smaller surfaces, they will exert greater pressure against the insides of a container. The lungs and vocal tract are just such containers.

The molecules comprising any substance, including gases, tend not to bounce around infinitely, but rather tend ultimately to slow down and cool off. This is the famous *principle of entropy*, which posits that if the molecules can reach a less active restful state, they will.

If and when they do reach this restful state, molecules no longer have the potential to do work, and the energy of any system in which they are contained decreases. Entropy would not be so good for us, because the universe, as we know it, would no longer exist. Fortunately for us, that state is a long way off.

Meanwhile, if those molecules can get to a larger volume, one in which they can assume a more comfortable proximity with other molecules, they will go right there. For gases, the desired volume is huge. On Earth, the result is that gases will always flow from conditions of higher pressure to conditions of lower pressure. This principle is known as the *Second Law of Thermodynamics*, or *Clausius' Law*, and it is the explanation for the flow of gases in and out of the respiratory system that accompanies changing respiratory volumes.

RESPIRATORY PRESSURES

Since air flows and behaves in certain ways, it is considered to be a *fluid* medium. Respiratory function for speech or metabolism depends on air flow, and this flow is accomplished by changes in pressures. Changes in pressures are, in turn, accomplished by changing volumes in pulmonary, thoracic, and abdominal cavities. Accordingly, pressures that affect respiration are called *alveolar pressure, pleural pressure,* and *abdominal pressure.*

ALVEOLAR PRESSURE

Alveolar pressure is air pressure within the lungs, particularly within the millions of alveolar sacks at the very ends of the bronchial tree branches. It is the air pressure we think of when we discuss air flow from lower lung volumes to higher, environmental volumes. Blom (2004) estimated normal alveolar pressure to be about 392 pascals (Pa).

Ochs and his colleagues (2004) counted between 274 and 790 million alveoli in the lungs of six samples, depending upon the size of the person. Even within the smallest person, this many alveoli produce an effective force. Pulmonary alveoli are stretched by the work of inspiratory muscles and sometimes, are compressed by the effects of expiratory muscles on the pleural spaces. They return to their pre-stretched shapes due to their own elastance, the property of a deformed object to return to its original shape, the fluid tension of a surfactant produced by type II cells in the alveoli, and the elastance of surrounding tissues. In any case, this causes a constant, rhythmic change in their volumes for tidal ventilation and a controlled volume change for speech.

PLEURAL PRESSURE

Pleural pressure is the internal pressure of the shallow layer of fluid between the parietal and visceral pleural membranes. Interpleural fluid is liquid formed from vessels in the visceral pleural membranes, and it flows from the apex of each lung to its base (Albertine, Wiener-Kronish, & Straub, 1984; Miserocchi, 1997). Like all liquids or gases in a thermodynamic system, pleural fluid flows from high pressure to low pressure. When the outer, parietal pleural membrane expands, it creates a larger volume in the interpleural space, lowering the fluid pressure of the interpleural fluid. This causes the visceral pleura to move closer to the parietal pleura, as a means of pressure equalization. Variations in interpleural fluid pressures mirror changes in alveolar pressures. Resting intrapleural pressures vary according to lung volume between approximately -196 Pa and -1,471 Pa. (Blom, 2004). Note that pressure outside the lungs (but still in the thorax) must be slightly negative with respect to pressure inside the lungs in order to keep the lungs and their alveolar spaces open.

ABDOMINAL PRESSURE

Mechanical pressure in the abdomen is applied superiorly against the thoracic tissues. It is created by the presence of the masses of abdominal contents and by muscular forces, and it varies with changes in the breather's posture by the acceleration of gravity. If the breather is upright, in anatomical position, the tendency of the diaphragm to be attracted to the parietal pleura as well as to the abdominal contents will tend to pull the abdominal contents superiorly as it also pulls the diaphragm inferiorly. If the breather is supine, gravity will force the abdominal contents down, towards the spine; laterally, to the body wall, pelvis, and thorax; and superiorly, toward the thorax.

Given the many possibilities for postural variations, including upper and lower limb excursions, abdominal pressure varies accordingly. Hodges and Gandevia (2000) found changes in abdominal and diaphragmatic pressures during quiet breathing between approximately 804 Pa (±127) and 1,353 Pa (±216) respectively, depending upon limb and spinal movement fluctuations.

Changes in abdominal pressure, then, affect the forces necessary to achieve a desired air flow for speech. This can become an important consideration in cases where an individual is bed-bound or has other postural concerns.

RELAXATION PRESSURE

Relaxation pressure is the inherent mechanical pressure to return lungs to the neutral resting state, not influenced by active muscular forces. It is created by the natural elastic tendency of the lungs, thoracic skeleton, and other thoracic tissues to return to a neutral state after having been stretched. It should be obvious, then, that relaxation pressure varies according to the phase of the respiratory cycle. In simple terms, relaxation pressures are negative during the expiratory phase and positive during the inspiratory phase. This has been established for many years. Rahn, Otis, Chadwick, & Fenn (1946) estimated relaxation pressures varying from about -3723 to +4903 Pa, depending upon the respiratory cycle phase.

PHYSICS OF RESPIRATION

The function of the respiratory system in speech is to provide a flowing column of air. When this air is restricted or impeded by the articulation of vocal tract structures, the kinetic energy inherent in the flowing gas is applied to creating one or two of three acoustic sources. These sources are the familiar phonatory source, fricative source, and plosive source.

The flow of gas in respiration depends, in part, on *Boyle's Law* (Boyle, 1662). This principle of gas physics relates gas pressure to its volume and states, "The volume of a fixed amount of gas maintained at a constant temperature is inversely proportional to the pressure of that gas." This principle can be expressed by the formula $P = 1/V$, with P meaning pressure and V meaning volume.

INSPIRATION

In tidal respiration, contraction of inspiratory muscles expands the thorax, sequentially increasing the volumes of the pleural cavities, the lungs, and alveoli and, thus, decreasing the pressure of the gas within. The pressure differential between the environment and the alveolar interiors draws additional gas into the enlarged alveolar spaces by the effects of Clausius' law, by which gases in high pressure regions will tend to flow into regions of lower pressure if they can. Relaxation of inspiratory muscles allows the natural respiratory system recoil forces to take over, and forces air out as pleural cavities, lungs, and alveolar space volumes decrease, subsequently increasing the pressure of the gas within and causing expiration. One may further reduce pulmonic volume and push additional air out of the thorax

if needed, but most of the time, relaxation pressures are sufficient.

Active muscular contraction expands the thorax during inspiration for either tidal or speech breathing. The primary muscles of inspiration are the *diaphragm*, located between the thorax and the abdomen, and the 11 paired *intercostal muscles*, located between the ribs.

Diaphragmatic movement increases the superior-inferior dimension of the thorax through flattening the dome shaped inferior thoracic margin. Costal movement is more complex, and has two main vectors (directions). Movements of the first six pairs of ribs and the sternum occur in a primarily anterior/superior direction. Such movement is sometimes referred to as *pump handle* movement. Ribs 7 to 10 move in a lateral and superior direction, sometimes described as *bucket handle* movement. The last two pairs of ribs, 11 and 12, are *floating* ribs, and do not play much of a role in breathing.

Respiration for speech requires controlled application of flowing gas pressure to the vocal tract. Since long utterances depend upon the sustained flow of air through the vocal tract, muscles of inspiration are usually active during speech in order to keep thoracic recoil forces under control. In this way, the thorax does not contract too quickly and does not expel necessary gas too soon. Expiratory muscles, and even secondary or accessory muscles, are available when an individual is exerted or when extended flow duration is desired for speaking long utterances.

LUNG VOLUME, AIR FLOW, AND ALVEOLAR PRESSURE

The key factor in determining respiratory airflow is the changing volumes in the approximately 274,000,000 to 790,000,000 tiny alveolar spaces within both lungs (Ochs et al., 2004). As lung alveolar volume increases during inspiration, alveolar pressure decreases (increases negatively), and then returns to zero when the lungs have pulled in their maximum volumes. Airflow, the rate of air in or out of the system, mirrors alveolar pressure. It increases negatively (meaning air flows into the system rather than out of the system), then ceases when maximum desired volume is reached. Alveolar volume decreases during expiration. Alveolar pressure increases positively, and then returns to zero at minimum volume. As you might expect, airflow does the same.

RESPIRATORY FORCE BALANCE IN SPEECH

During respiratory activity, there is a tension or balance between muscular forces and thoracic relaxation forces. Whether for tidal breathing or for speech purposes, muscular and relaxation forces combine and balance to achieve the desired flow. The easiest, least effortful approach is to allow relaxation forces to do all the work. This is the most common pattern in tidal breathing. After all, energy has already been expended and stored in the *recoil spring* of the thorax. Speech breathing is a different matter, because the desired flow is subject to the idiosyncrasies of the speaker. Muscular forces may take over at any point, such as when the speaker decides to stop speaking or when the speaker decides to change the amplitude or duration of the utterance.

We have identified the key quantity in determining the air flow during speech as *alveolar pressure variation*. Alveolar pressure variation, in turn, depends on the balance between muscular and relaxation forces. When alveolar pressure is less than relaxation pressure, then the inspiratory muscles are in control. If alveolar pressure is greater than relaxation pressure, then expiratory muscles are in control. When alveolar pressure is equal to relaxation pressure, then no muscular forces are involved. Of course this creates a very complex set of parameters, for each alveolar pressure in speech demands a different muscular pressure at each lung volume.

In clinical work, it is important that the speaker's posture, health, coordination, and strength be considered when assessing the capabilities of respiratory support for speech. Parameters of respiratory functions have essential implications for the fluency, amplitude, duration, and stability of speech.

REFERENCES

Albertine, K. H., Wiener-Kronish, J. P., & Straub, N. C. (1984). The structure of the parietal pleura and its relationship to pleural liquid dynamics in sheep. *The Anatomical Record, 208*, 401-409.

Backman, H., Lindberg, A., Sovijärvi, A., Larsson, K., Lundbäck B., & Rönmark, E. (2015). Evaluation of the global lung function initiative 2012 reference values for spirometry in a Swedish population sample *BMC Pulmonary Medicine, 15*(26). doi: 10.1186/s12890-015-0022-2

Binazzi, B., Lanini, B., Bianchi, R., Romagnoli, I., Nerini, M., Gigliotti, F., Scano, G. (2006). Breathing pattern and kinematics in normal subjects during speech, singing and loud whispering. *Acta Physiologica, 186*, 233-246.

Blom, J. A. (2004). *Monitoring of respiration and circulation*. Boca Raton, FL: CRC Press.

Eklund, R. (2008). Pulmonic ingressive phonation: Diachronic and synchronic characteristics, distribution and function in animal and human sound production and in human speech. *Journal of the International Phonetic Association, 38*, 235-324.

Hodges, P. W., & Gandevia, S. C. (2000). Changes in intra-abdominal pressure during postural and respiratory activation of the human diaphragm. *Journal of Applied Physiology, 89*, 967-976.

Miserocchi, G. (1997). Physiology and pathophysiology of pleural fluid turnover. *The European Respiratory Journal 10*, 219-25.

Ochs, M., Nyengaard, J. R., Jung, A., Knudsen, L., Voigt, M., Wahlers, T., et al., (2004). The number of alveoli in the human lung. *American Journal of Respiratory Critical Care Medicine, 169*, 120-124.

Rahn H., Otis A. B., Chadwick E., & Fenn W. O. (1946). The pressure-volume diagram of the thorax and lung. *American Journal of Physiology, 146*, 161-178.

Part 2: Phonation and Speech

GOAL

Examine phonation as an aspect of speech science.

OBJECTIVES

- Recognize the phonetic importance of phonation.
- Recognize phonatory importance in prosody.
- Recognize parameters of syllabic stress.
- Distinguish voicing from whispering.
- Relate subglottal pressure magnitudes to phonatory amplitude.
- Recognize phases of glottal triangular wave.
- Relate Bernoulli's principle to phonation.
- Recognize the mucoviscoelastic theory of phonation.
- Distinguish jitter from shimmer.
- Distinguish among laryngeal postures used for whispering, falsetto, glottal plosive, pulsation, and laryngealization.

• • • • • • •

The function of the phonatory mechanism in speech is to create and modulate three acoustic sources, the most frequently used of which is commonly called the *voice*. Speech scientists call this source the *phonatory source*. The phonatory source can assume various spectral qualities through manipulation of the vocal folds, depending upon the desires of the speaker. The voice is employed in production of most speech sounds, by far. In fact, it is easier to count the phonemes that don't use the phonatory source than it is to count those that do use it. Thus, it accompanies production of all vowels, approximants, and nasals, and about half the obstruent consonants. In obstruent consonant production, under normal circumstances, the phonatory source serves as a phonemic marker, distinguishing voiced and voiceless cognates and, therefore, meaning in minimal pair words such as "Pig," and "Big."

The parameters of phonation in speech vary quite a bit with changes in suprasegmental characteristics. Quantifiable prosodic parameters include *fundamental frequency, intensity, spectrum*, and *durations* of the voice source. These, you will recall, are perceived by listeners (and, one would hope, speakers) as *pitch, loudness, quality*, and *length*. For example, phonatory frequency, perceived as vocal pitch, usually increases at the ends of

sentences asking questions, and decreases at the ends of statements. Frequency, amplitude, quality, and even duration change with variations in syllabic stress, emphasis, and intonation. These, as you can readily see, are consciously or unconsciously associated with the communicative intent of an utterance.

Physically, increased syllabic stress is manifested by increases in duration and amplitude of the syllabic nucleus, and may also involve increased fundamental frequency. The saying goes, "Stressed segments are longer and stronger." Emphasis and intonation are dependent upon the pragmatic circumstances under which a syllable or group of syllables will be used.

ALTERNATIVE GLOTTAL POSTURES

Producing sounds with the vocal folds is called *phonation*, and all sounds produced by action of the vocal folds are called *phonatory*. This means that whispering is a form of phonation, even though the whispered voice and the normal voice are produced in different ways. A normal phonatory source is called *modal voicing*, so named because a statistical mode is the most frequently observed value, while a whispered phonatory source is

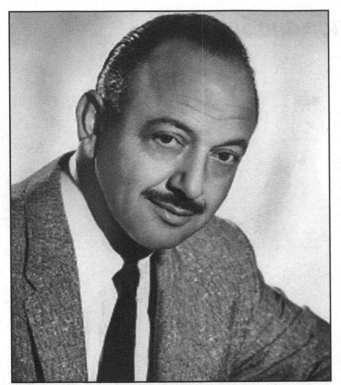

Figure 6.2-1. Mel Blanc (1908–1989) was a gifted vocal artist, best known for his characterizations of Looney Tunes cartoon characters. According to a newspaper story in 1988, Blanc claimed that a physician told him his pharyngeal musculature was similar to that of an opera singer.

called, appropriately enough, *whispering*. There is also *breathy* phonation, *creaky* or *pulsed* phonation, and *falsetto* phonation, to name a few more.

It may come as a surprise to some that the larynx is extremely flexible, and a gifted speaker is able to produce a wide range of vocal productions depending largely upon which muscles are brought into play (see Figure 6.2-1). Modal phonation is just one of the actions the larynx performs during speech. When a speaker configures muscles and other tissues in a particular manner, for phonation or other speech purposes, the speaker is said to be assuming a posture. Alternate glottal postures can have a perceptible effect on the output of the larynx. Some of these postures may be phonemic.

Whispering is produced with the anterior portion of the glottis adducted and a small aperture formed at the posterior end. Air flows through this constriction, producing the *glottal fricative* as an aperiodic continuous acoustic source, used phonemically as a consonant, /h/. There is a voiced cognate of the glottal fricative, produced with a form of breathy phonation. The phonetic symbol for the voiced glottal fricative is /ɦ/.

Falsetto voice, a phonatory source of very high frequency relative to a speaker's modal voice, is produced by tensing the lateral part of the glottis and allowing the medial part to vibrate. This effectively lowers the mass of the folds, making it possible for them to move at greater speed, shortening the glottal cycle period and resulting in a higher pitch.

The *glottal plosive* is formed by trapping air beneath the glottis and releasing it suddenly. Syllables released by vowels may be said to have a glottal plosive for a releaser. An older, but frequently encountered, name for the glottal plosive is the *glottal stop*.

Vocal fry, or *pulsation*, is produced by voicing with a very low fundamental frequency. The frequency of a pulsed voice is around 20 to 90 Hertz (Hz). This type of phonation is often observed when the speaker is using the lower end of his or her pitch range. Related to pulsation is *laryngealization*. This kind of phonation occurs often at the end of declarative utterances when the glottal frequency decreases rapidly.

VOICING PHYSIOLOGY

Sound generation in voicing is accomplished by sustained, nearly periodic, cyclical valving of pulmonic air. To make this happen, air must be flowing outward from the trachea and the vocal folds are adducted, or approximated just tight enough to meet the speaker's needs (see Figure 6.2-2). These needs depend upon how much force is required to just barely resist the force of air built up by the contracting thorax. Vocal folds must be adducted with enough force, or *medial compression*, to allow air impounded below to build up pressure sufficient to create a voice of the desired amplitude.

The force of the flowing air and the force of vocal fold adduction is manipulated by the speaker according to the pragmatics of the speaking situation. If the speaker is going to use a normal, conversational voice, then the thorax just relaxes, using the combined forces provided by the natural tendency of high pressure gas to flow out, the spring-like tendency of the ribs and other thoracic tissues to return to their normal positions, and the tendency of the lungs to pull inward. If a speaker wishes to add the energy of a louder voice to an utterance, the force of expiration will increase, and the force of adduction will increase accordingly.

Whether or not the speaker contracts the muscles of expiration, an increase of air pressure inferior to the adducted vocal folds is necessary to provide energy for the acoustic source. The pressure of the air below the glottis is called *subglottal pressure*. The greater the magnitude of subglottal pressure, the greater will

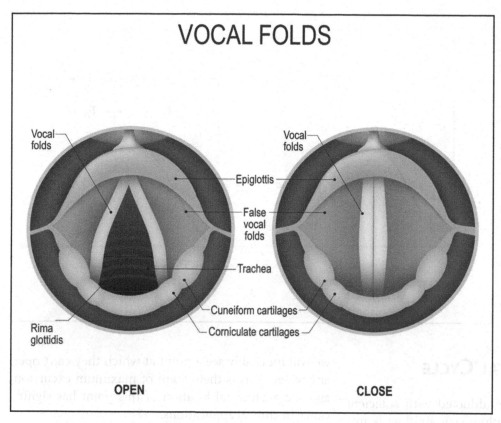

VOCAL FOLDS

Vocal folds — Epiglottis — Vocal folds

— False vocal folds

— Trachea

— Cuneiform cartilages

Rima glottidis — Corniculate cartilages

OPEN — CLOSE

Figure 6.2-2. Slightly abducted vocal folds. (Designua/Shutterstock.com)

be the subsequent sound pressure level of the output (Ladefoged & McKinney, 1963). Further, subglottal pressure is increased by increasing the force by which air is expired in combination with resisting the force of expired air with the opposing force of increased glottal adduction.

At some point, however, audible speech demands that subglottal pressure must force the adducted vocal folds apart, and when it does, the air will flow out through the glottal opening, displacing the adducted vocal folds. If the folds are adducted for normal vocal amplitudes, about 60 dB SPL for conversational speech, then subglottal pressure builds to a normal level. Ladefoged and his colleagues (1963) estimated that for voicing to begin in their experimental subjects, subglottal pressure must reach 588 Pa [volumes converted to SI], and that sustained voicing in running speech required subglottal pressure to be maintained at 680 to 980 Pa. For louder levels of voicing, greater pressure is required. So, of course, is greater glottal adduction force, since subglottal pressure has to be resisted in order for it to increase to sufficient magnitudes.

The sound of the voice is created because higher pressure subglottal air, compared to lower pressure supraglottal air, means subglottal gas molecules are pushed closer together and are more excited. They want to expand and equalize. High pressure air forces the vocal folds apart and passes through the glottis, exciting the adjacent air in a rhythmic series of pulses, and creating the acoustic phonatory source. It is important to note that the sound of the voice is not the sound of the vocal folds slapping together like clapping hands, although that kind of contact might contribute minimally. It is mostly the sound of high-pressure air pulses propagating pressure changes, not unlike the sound of a balloon popping, but closer to the sound of 120 to 250 balloons popping every second, depending upon the perceived pitch of the voice. The same thing happens with a small gasoline engine, except a different gas is involved. The sound you hear is the sound of high pressure gas exiting the exhaust pipe in rapid pulses.

If the excited air puffs occurred in regular sequence, without change over time, we could say the sound is periodic. However, the vibrations of the voice are not truly periodic, since they don't have a regular frequency. Small variations in neuromuscular control and the balance between muscular and mechanical forces make it impossible for a human being to produce a perfectly periodic glottal wave, not to mention intentional changes imposed by the prosodic aspects of the speaker's utterance. Instead, the phonatory source is properly called *quasi-periodic*, or *almost periodic*.

Figure 6.2-3. Study the two cycles of a typical glottal flow waveform above. The variables shown are as follows: **Tp**—the part of the glottal cycle in which airflow rate is increasing (thus, the slope of the curve is going upward during this time). Think of "p" for positive; **Tn**—the part of the glottal cycle in which airflow rate is decreasing (downward slope in the curve). Here, "n" represents negative; **To**—the length of time during each cycle in which air is flowing (i.e., the folds are open); **T**—the total duration of each vibrational cycle; **uo**—the average rate of airflow; **uac**—the maximum rate of flow. Visit http://www.ncvs.org/ncvs/tutorials/voiceprod/tutorial/graphing.html for more information about the figure. (Reprinted by permission from author Ingo R. Titze from *Principles of Voice Production*, Chapter 5, p. 127, NCVS, 2000)

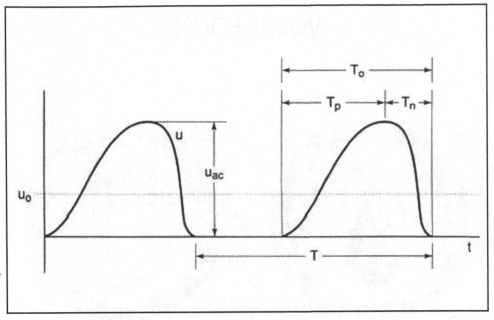

THE GLOTTAL CYCLE

Once the vocal folds are adducted with sufficient medial compression, and pulmonary air flow is impeded, air pressure below the glottis increases. At a critical magnitude imposed by the muscular and elastic forces present, the membranous portion of the glottis gives way, and a series of cyclic openings and closing of the glottis begins, continuing until the speaker stops it. This, in turn, creates an egressive series of pressure changes in the vocal tract that a listener perceives as a voice.

The pressure changes produced at the glottis are described as changes in *volume velocity*. Volume velocity is rate of air flow through the glottis, and it is easy to appreciate that this rate is greatest when the glottis is opened to its fullest extent, gradually rising to a peak and falling off as the glottis closes. The formula for volume velocity is air flow divided by acoustic impedance, meaning that the quantity is greatest when impedance is least. Graphic depictions of volume velocity changes are visually very similar to graphic depictions of glottal area changes during phonatory cycles.

Just like any other cyclic phenomenon, the glottal cycle has phases. A glottal cycle can begin at any degree of opening and closing, or any phase. We can imagine looking down on a cycling glottis from the entrance to the larynx, and we will see it opening and closing. If we start counting at the very instant the glottis begins to open, calling that phase zero degrees, and follow the cycle as the vocal folds move farther and farther apart,

we will inevitably see a point at which they can't open any wider. This is their point of maximum excursion, and the anatomical location of this point has significance in clinical applications.

As soon as the vocal folds reach the point of maximum excursion, the glottis begins to close, and the vocal folds steadily move closer together until they touch, or nearly touch in modal phonation, and the glottis is effectively closed. If phonation is to continue, the glottis will remain closed until sufficient air pressure exists beneath to force it open again. At this instant, the glottis begins to open again, and we are back to zero degrees, ready to begin another glottal cycle. After one cycle, the process repeats itself until the speaker either decides to stop phonating, or runs out of air, or both.

It is noteworthy that the vocal folds do not necessarily have to create a complete closure at the glottis to produce a phonatory acoustic source. However, the more space existing between the approximated vocal folds, the more turbulent air is created and the "breathier" the voice sounds.

Voice physiologists have analyzed the glottal cycle to more fully understand phonation, and new information is gained regularly (see Figure 6.2-3). On a fundamental level, there are two phases to the cycle: a *closed phase* and an *open phase*. For a modal voice, as you might imagine, the folds are touching each other along their entire medial borders during the closed phase, and they are apart to some degree during the open phase.

During the closed phase of phonation, the vocal folds are loosely adducted by the forces provided by muscles of glottal adduction. Air pressure produced by relaxation of the muscles of inspiration (or, sometimes contraction of the muscles of expiration) builds up inferior to the vocal folds and forces them open. As soon as there is the least opening between the folds, they are said to be in the open phase.

The open phase can be broken down further into two parts: an *opening phase* during which the folds are moving away from the midline under pressure from pulmonic air, and a *closing phase*, during which the folds are moving back toward the midline. During a typical glottal cycle, the opening phase is longer than the closing phase.

A graph of glottal area changes over time during cycling helps visualize the cycle and understand it better. As the glottis opens, its area increases, and as it closes, its area decreases. Note that there are no negative values since the glottis cannot be closed more than fully closed, or have an area less than zero. Since the graph is a function of vocal fold tissue as it moves over time, it will look like a very poorly drawn triangle. For this reason, the glottal wave is sometimes said to be triangular, even though it barely qualifies as a triangle. It is called triangular because it has no negative values. Although the exact parameters depend upon the speaker, frequency, and amplitude, the open phase is longer than the closed phase, occupying about 87% of the entire cycle. This means that during phonation, the glottis is open far longer than it is closed, and once opening begins, it takes longer for the vocal folds to reach maximum excursion than it does for them to close.

Vocal fold vibratory frequency depends, of course, upon how fast the vocal folds move. The faster they can move, the more vibrations can occur each second, and the higher the perceived pitch of the voice will be. Given equal driving forces, lighter vocal folds (vocal folds with less mass) can move faster than heavier ones. Pulling a given vocal fold tighter decreases its mass per unit length, making it vibrate faster. Greater vocal fold masses produce lower pitches.

We have maintained that vocal fold cycles are not perfectly uniform, meaning that there are quantifiable variations between cycles. Cycle-to-cycle variations in vocal fold vibratory frequency (or period) are called *jitter*. Tiny and large changes in muscular tension, and the balance among relaxation pressure, muscle pressure, and adduction pressures in the thorax and larynx, all serve to cause variations in vibratory frequency. Jitter may be noticeable or not, and may be voluntary or involuntary. Involuntary jitter is, of course unavoidable. Abnormally large jitter may be an early diagnostic

sign of neuromuscular dysfunction, and is of interest to health professionals, including speech-language pathologists. This can be tracked with a speech spectrograph.

Speakers can vary amplitude as well as frequency of their vocal vibrations, and amplitude variations are called *shimmer*. Changes in phonatory amplitude accompany changing subglottal pressure along with changes in medial compression forces. Until the middle of the last century, it was thought that the further apart the vocal folds are blown by pulmonic air pressure—that is, the greater the amplitude of displacement—the louder the voice. Recent research has reported, however, that this is only the case for some speakers. For others, there is no difference in the distance of maximum vocal fold displacement. This would suggest that variations in volume velocity do not always reflect changes in the glottal area. It is the magnitude of air pressure that is critical.

The mechanism for changing glottal cycle amplitude depends upon the coordinated action of the muscles of respiration and the muscles of glottal adduction. Respiratory forces increase subglottal pressure, but glottal adductors must increase vocal fold resistance in order to allow that pressure to increase. If we increase the force of pulmonic air by contracting the muscles of expiration, we can increase subglottal pressure. But the loosely adducted folds will simply give away if we don't accompany the pulmonic force with increased adductive force. With increases in subglottal air pressure comes increases in aerodynamic forces that bring the vocal folds back to the midline. Thus, a louder voice—that is, one generated with greater sound pressure—is produced with greater muscular forces and with greater aerodynamic forces. Research has demonstrated that acoustic intensity is related to the third or fourth power of subglottal pressure, or that doubling subglottal pressure results in nine to 12 decibels of intensity increase (Ladefoged & McKinney, 1963).

It should be clear by now that phonation is largely dependent upon air pressure management. To set the folds in motion, sufficient air pressure below the adducted glottis must exist. A typical magnitude of subglottal air pressure for sustained speech is 800 Pa (Zhang, 2016). The onset of phonation, or *voice onset*, is relatively easy to understand. However, what forces make the vocal folds vibrate in succession and maintain that vibration?

The physics of phonatory cycling has been a subject of debate for many years, and the discussion continues. The *myoelastic-aerodynamic* principle of phonation has been an accepted explanation to sustained vocal fold vibratory forces from about 1950 to the present. More recent study has cast doubts on the adequacy of such a simple explanation for such a complex cyclic movement (Zhang, 2016). Briefly stated, the myoelastic-aerodynamic principle of phonation asserts that vocal fold vibration is maintained by the combined actions of muscular and aerodynamic forces (van den Berg, 1958). The myoelastic part of the principle means that the vocal folds are held together by constant tonic muscular pressure until the speaker decides to stop phonating. The aerodynamic principle is that the folds are forced apart by increased subglottal air pressure and brought back together by the *Bernoulli effect.*

The Bernoulli effect describes the lower pressure created by relative increases in the velocity of a liquid medium, such as the air in the vocal tract. As applied to phonation, air flowing through the glottis near the surfaces of the vocal folds has a slightly greater distance to cover than air flowing straight up through the center. Since the air near the vocal folds and the air in the center must reach the same destination at the same time, the air near the vocal folds must move faster than the air in the center. This means the air closest to the vocal folds has a lower pressure than the air in the center, and this lower pressure tends to draw the vocal fold tissues centrally. The faster the air flows, the greater is the effect.

In essence, the Bernoulli effect is an expression of the law of conservation of energy or the first law of thermodynamics. You will recall that this principle holds that the total amount of available energy is stable in a closed system, and it is expressed as either potential energy or kinetic energy. Potential energy is energy that is stored, like that in compressed air, and kinetic energy is that which is in action, like flowing air. The gas closest to the vocal fold surface moves faster than that flowing through the center of the glottal opening, and this increased velocity of gas along the vocal fold surface trades potential energy for kinetic energy. Reducing potential energy is the same as reducing air pressure, so there is lower air pressure next to the vocal folds than there is in the middle of the glottis. The lower pressure sucks the fold back to the middle of the glottis, helping to close it during the glottal cycle.

Essential to the vibratory characteristics of the vocal folds is the fact that there are structural tissue differences in the leading (lower) edge of the focal folds and the trailing (upper) edge. These differences cause phase differentials between movements of the lower and upper glottal tissues, and alter the shape of the glottal aperture to optimize the airflow and tissue resiliency. The effect was described by Hiroto (1966) and called the muco-*viscoelastic aerodynamic* theory of phonation.

Hiroto's elaboration of the mucoviscoelastic properties of vocal folds opened the door to further explorations of vocal fold vibratory mechanics. In particular, vocal physiologists have taken a closer look at the mucoviscoelastic aspect of the mucoviscoelastic-aerodynamic principle. Titze (1975), Story (2015), Zhang (2016), and others have posited that the very heterogeneous, or anisotropic cohesive, nature of vocal fold tissues cause them to vibrate in different manners depending upon the anatomical location of the particular kind of tissue that is vibrating. However, ultimately and essentially, the entire vocal fold will vibrate in one or more synchronized cyclic patterns called *eigenmodes.* Differing vibratory characteristics in these eigenmodal cycles resonate with one another in much the same way as air in the vocal tract, amplifying their vibratory energy as it is transferred from the pressure of subglottal air. In this manner, Zhang (2016) and others have posited that the very heterogeneity of vocal fold structure leads to their vibration quasi-independently of the air stream, minimizing the role of the Bernoulli effect through the amplifying resonation of their molecular structures.

An interesting and practically important aspect of the mucoviscoelastic aerodynamic principle of phonation is that there is a balance between the effects of muscle tension and aerodynamics in accomplishing the closing phase of the glottal cycle. Still, energy to create vocal fold vibration must have a source, and the possible sources of that energy are some combinations of the molecular forces of the vocal fold tissues, or the energy supplied through neuromuscular effort, or pneumatic energy supplied by the air stream. Thus, in speaking situations with diminished air flow, such as when expiratory volumes are nearly depleted, muscular tension can compensate to accomplish glottal closing by either adding medial compressive forces or by altering the laminar nature of the folds themselves. There are limits to the efficiency of this tact, and since muscular effort is harder to sustain than airflow, the result can be vocal fatigue. The best bet for a speaker seeking to minimize vocal fatigue is to re-inflate the lungs to mid-volumes and continue using airflow as the principle force for glottal closing.

Other laryngeal changes occur in the glottal cycle with changes in amplitude. Assuming a nearly constant frequency, increased amplitude means that the vocal folds close with more force, because they are under more Bernoulli effect and under more muscular tension, and they stay closed a little longer because they slammed together so hard and because they are under more muscle tension.

All this high-speed contact might have a deleterious effect on the tissues of the vocal folds, wouldn't you think? Try clapping your hands real hard for about a minute. What happens? Well, the vocal folds are probably tenderer than your hands.

Increased subglottal pressure can also be accompanied by increased frequency measurements. This is probably because the speaker often, but not always, reflexively increases vocal fold tension as subglottal pressure increases, tightening the vocal ligaments in the process. Notice the slight increase in vocal pitch that often occurs during stressed syllable utterances.

Phonatory functions not only provide the major acoustic energy source for speech, but also provide the ability to add inflection, tone, and even interest and music to the signal. It is no wonder that voice science is such a fertile field for scholars and practitioners interested in speech.

REFERENCES

Broad, D. (1973) in Minifie, F., Hixon, T., & Williams, F. (1973). *Normal aspects of speech hearing and language*. Englewood Cliffs, N.J.: Prentice Hall.

Harmetz, A. (1988, November 24). Man of a thousand voices, speaking literally. *New York Times*. Retrieved from http://www.nytimes.com/1988/11/24/arts/man-of-a-thousand-voices-speaking-literally.html

Hiroto, P. (1966). Patho-physiology of the larynx from the standpoint of vocal mechanism [in Japanese]. *Practa Otologica Kyoto, 59*, 229-292.

Ladefoged, P. & McKinney, N. P. (1963). Loudness, sound pressure, and subglottal pressure in speech. *The Journal of the Acoustical Society of America 35*, 454-460. doi: http://dx.doi.org/10.1121/1.1918503

Story, B. H. (2015). Mechanisms of voice production. In M.A. Redford (Ed.), *The handbook of speech production* (pp. 34-57). Hoboken, NJ: John Wiley & Sons, Inc.

Titze, I. R., & Strong, W. J. (1975). Normal modes in vocal cord tissues. *Journal of the Acoustical Society of America, 57*, 736-744.

van den Berg, J. (1958). Myoelastic-aerodynamic theory of voice production. *Journal of Speech and Hearing Research, 1*, 227-244.

Zhang, Z. (2016). Mechanics of human voice production and control. *The Journal of the Acoustical Society of America, 140*, 2614–2635. http://doi.org/10.1121/1.4964509

Part 3: Articulation and Speech

GOAL

Examine elementary normal speech articulatory processes.

OBJECTIVES

○ Distinguish among speech articulatory muscle groups.
○ Recognize three sound sources for speech.
○ Distinguish among voice onset times (VOTs) for tense and lax initial obstruent consonants.
○ Recognize four sources of allophonic variation.
○ Distinguish among syllable boundaries and nuclei.
○ Distinguish between two types of articulatory juncture.

• • • • • •

MOTOR SPEECH PROCESSES

The term *motor speech* is often used to describe the muscular actions employed by a speaker to change the shape and patency of the vocal tract in such a way as to change its resonating characteristics and alter the air flow through it, creating the sounds of meaningful speech. In this sense, motor speech actions are considered apart from higher-level psycholinguistic processes. Successful speech articulation is the result of coordinated and precise muscular actions of mobile vocal tract structures acting in concert with the respiratory system, including the larynx, and, of course, the motor support of the nervous system. Speech articulation is at its best when a listener's attention is fully devoted to the linguistic content of the speaker's message rather than the speaker's manner of speaking.

Vocal tract structures can be categorized as *mobile* or *fixed*. To produce the sounds of speech, a speaker moves the mobile structures in relationship to one another or to relatively immoveable fixed structures to effect the motor aspects of speech articulation. Mobile structures include the lips, tongue, and pharyngeal muscles, including those of the velopharyngeal sphincter and glottis. Fixed structures include the teeth, superior alveolar ridge, and the so-called *hard palate*, formed by processes of the maxilla and palatine bones and their soft tissue coverings.

The concept of dynamic function is essential to understanding speech articulation, for it is rare that anyone speaks in single, static speech postures. During speech articulation, moving vocal tract structures—such as the lips, tongue, velopharyngeal sphincter, mandible, and vocal folds—act by moving in juxtaposition to each other and to fixed vocal tract structures, such as the teeth, superior alveolar ridge, palate, and velum. In this sense, speech can be imagined as a dance, or flowing sequence of movements, subject to inertia, mistakes, and self-corrections. When the flow of movements is smooth and uninterrupted, speech is *fluent*. The flow can be, and often is, interrupted, and the speech becomes *dysfluent*. Most speakers and listeners accept a modicum of dysfluency as normal and pay it little attention. In fact, speakers who are perfectly fluent are usually the likes of multimedia announcers who have rehearsed their lines.

On a strictly physiological level, and forgetting, for the moment, the thoughts, motivations, personal idiosyncrasies, and ideas of central language processing, the movements of vocal tract structures can be understood as purely motor speech functions. We have seen earlier that the entire motor system, including that part used in speaking, is a complex network of pyramidal (voluntary) and extrapyramidal (involuntary) neurons. Speech movements begin as voluntary neural impulses propagated by upper motor neurons in the precentral cerebral cortical gyri, pre-preprogrammed and refined by the other levels of the motor system, and monitored by unconscious and conscious sensory neural impulses received in central sensory centers.

Coordination of speech muscle groups is essential to normal speech articulation. These muscle groups act in concert, with increasing precision timing and strength, and it takes a speaker time and experience to do so well.

Speech muscle groups include respiratory muscles, acting in a concerted interplay of inspiratory and expiratory groups. Phonatory muscles involved in speech are primarily the intrinsic laryngeal muscles, although extrinsic muscles are brought into play for special purposes. Facial muscles play a key role in articulation of labial consonants and rounded vowels. Some approximants, such as /r/, and the fricatives /ʃ/ and /ʒ/ are also quite often articulated with accompanying lip rounding. Articulation of most phonemes would be impossible without the contractions and movements of the lingual muscles and muscles of mandibular elevation, and of course, we can't discuss articulatory muscle groups without including the muscles that activate the velopharyngeal sphincter and other muscles of the pharynx.

These muscle groups function in concert, in controlled, rhythmic patterns. The timing and intensity of contractions is tuned with experience. One of the basic rationales in speech therapy is to provide such experiences.

But speech articulation isn't just about muscular contractions. Feedback is extremely important. In some ways, feedback places the speaker in the position of the listener, as she or he listens to and feels her or his own speech. The auditory feedback signal delivered to a speaker is not quite the same as that received by a listener. Differences in the acoustic wave that the speaker hears and that the listener hears are created by differences in the vibrating medium: the listener hears the source vibration through the air medium, while the speaker hears the source propagated through the bone medium and air medium.

Other forms of feedback are available only to the speaker. Speaker feedback is also tactile, with the speaker feeling the movements and contacts of the articulators as speech progresses (Tourville, Reilly, & Gunther, 2008). The speaker can change or self-correct the spoken output at will according to the feedback. Of course, feedback may also be visual, depending upon whether the speaker can see the listener.

SPEECH SOUND SOURCES

Speech articulation is the speaker's effort to create intelligible and distinctive utterances by using vocal tract structures to manipulate the spectral characteristics of combinations of three acoustic sources: the phonatory source, the fricative source and the plosive source. The phonatory source is a quasiperiodic, continuous sound; the fricative source is an aperiodic, continuous sound; and the plosive source is an aperiodic, transient sound.

These sources will, of course, usually be propagated through media of air or bone, depending upon whether the listener is also the speaker, in what's called a *feed-back loop*. The sources may also be propagated over electroacoustic media. How closely the propagation media duplicate the original signal is crucial to the viability of those media for efficient communication.

The phonatory source, also known as the voice, is the only acoustic source for all phonemes except the voiceless (*tense* or *surd*) obstruent consonants. Thus, the phonatory source is the major acoustic phenomenon in vowels, approximants, and nasals. These phonemes rely on variations of the spectral characteristics of the phonatory input source as a means of categorical discrimination by the listener. The articulatory postures are mostly open, being created by changes in the volumes of oral, pharyngeal, and labial cavities. Thus, there is effectively an infinite range of possible postures creating a wide variety of spectral variations in the phonatory source input spectrum.

The range of acceptable articulatory postures and subsequent spectral variations for each of the vowels is quite broad, explaining why vowels are seldom the targets of speech therapy. It also offers an explanation for why dialectical variations most often involve vowels. The IPA categorizes vowel articulation postures along a continuum of degrees and locations of maximum vocal tract constrictions created by tongue movements, and with most of the resonances subject to further modification by lip rounding. It displays these postures in a trapezoidal diagram known to phoneticians as the *vowel quadrilateral* (see Figure 6.3-1).

Using this chart as a guide, degree of vocal tract constriction ranges continuously from open to close, with the tongue held close to the roof of the mouth for close vowels, such as /i/, and low for open vowels, such as /a/ (see Figure 6.3-2). Location of vocal tract constriction is on a continuum from front to back. Front vowels are, thus, /e and /ɛ/, while back vowels include /o/ and /ɔ/. Varying degrees of lip rounding is a possible accompaniment for most of the vowel tongue postures, varying with the particular language. The degree of lip rounding is not specified on the IPA chart, but is, instead, indicated by a diacritical mark. In American English dialect, only the back series of vowels is rounded, with the degree of lip rounding becoming tighter as the tongue posture becomes closer, such as with the close back vowel /u/.

Approximant articulation may be imagined as being very similar to articulation of close vowels, with a major added distinctive perceptual cue of dynamic, ongoing spectral change or formant transition. True, formant transition is critical to normal-sounding speech

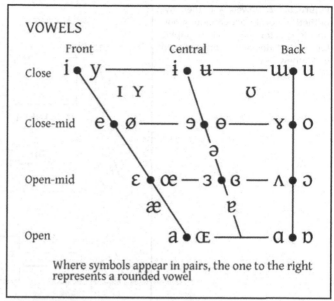

Figure 6.3-1. Vowel quadrilateral. https://www.internationalphoneticas-sociation.org/ ("Ipa-chart-vowels.png" by Grendelkhan, Nohat / used under CC BY-SA 3.0)

in most running speech, but in approximants /w/, /j/, and /r/, it is essential to categorical distinction and, in some cases, intelligibility. For these approximants, failure to move or "glide" the tongue or lips while moving directly to a vowel or other syllable nucleus results in their changing from syllable boundaries, or consonants, to syllable nuclei. The close relationship between vowels and approximants leaves perceptual confusion as a possibility and results in the often-heard articulatory confusions, such as among various manifestations of /r/, /w/, /ɝ or ɚ/, and /ɜ or ə/, or /l/ and /w/. An exception to this is the dental-alveolar-postalveolar lateral approximant, /l/, which can be held static as long as the speaker has the breath without compromising its categorical identity. Adding to the rich acoustic color palate of approximant articulation is the fact that some approximants are modified by lip rounding in certain phonetic contexts, and even /l/ is sometimes confused with /o/ as a dialectical or individual (*idiolectical*) variant.

The fricative and plosive sources are employed when the speaker articulates obstruent consonants, called, appropriately enough, fricatives and plosives. As we know, these aperiodic sources are combined with the phonatory source when the speaker articulates voiced obstruent consonants.

Articulatory possibilities are more discreet for the obstruent consonants than they are for vowels, making articulatory accuracy more critical for the speaker.

Figure 6.3-2. Vowels and their hypothetical vocal tract configurations, power spectra, and spectrographic formant relationships. (Image drawn by Mathew DeVore)

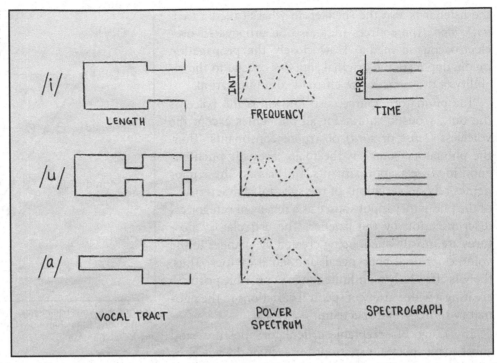

This makes plosives and fricatives a frequent target of speech therapy plans.

For the listener, categorical perception of obstruent consonants depends upon variations in the frequencies of high energy bands in the continuous spectra of aperiodic sound sources. These broad spectra range in frequency from less than 100 Hz to just over 20,000 Hz, with the greatest amplitudes in the region between 2,000 and 10,000 Hz, depending upon the vocal tract posture. Compared to the output for vowels, overall amplitudes of obstruent consonants are impeded by the relatively closed articulatory postures of these phonemes. High-frequency, low-amplitude output spectra may present a problem for listeners with high-frequency hearing loss, or for listeners in a noisy environment.

For obstruent consonants, the place of maximum vocal tract constriction is the place where the aperiodic acoustic sources are generated. Regions of high energy in the output spectra of obstruents are varied by moving the place of articulation forward to backward in the vocal tract, thereby moving the location of the sound source. This variability of source location is one obvious feature that distinguishes obstruent consonants from other types of speech sounds. The most anterior, or distal, source location along the length of the vocal tract tube for obstruent consonants is the bilabial location. Moving back, places of aperiodic source productions for English consonants are, in sequence, labiodental, dental, alveolar, postalveolar, palatal, velar, and glottal.

As the place of articulation, that is, the place of maximum vocal tract constriction, moves back from the bilabial to the glottal, the volume of the vocal tract cavity in front of the constriction increases. For the same reason, the volume of the cavity behind the constriction decreases. Thus, the volume of the cavity in front of the bilabial place of articulation has no volume, and the volume of the cavity behind the glottal place of constriction has no volume.

The volume of the cavity in front of the source has the most distinctive effect on the output spectrum of the obstruent consonant, since the focus of its energy is in that anterior direction. A smaller volume in front of the place of source production means bands in the higher frequency regions of the source spectrum have the greatest amplitudes. Larger volumes in front of the constriction distribute their high energy bands in the lower frequency regions.

Another source of spectral variation is lip rounding. Fricatives are often articulated with accompanying lip rounding just like vowels and approximants. Lip rounding extends the vocal tract slightly, creating additional volume in front of the constriction, and shifting energy to the lower bands of the continuous fricative spectrum. Perhaps the most frequently rounded fricative in English is the postalveolar fricative, /ʃ/, often used as a vocal gesture requesting silence. It is noteworthy that an almost universal gesture for, "Please be quiet," is placing a finger in front of the lips.

SYLLABLES

The syllable is the minimal motoric segment of speech, and it is by examining the natures of syllables that we find a good place to begin details of speech articulation processes. Syllables are much discussed, and most phoneticians seem to recognize one whey they see one. Unfortunately, there is no uniform definition of the concept, even though clinical practitioners spend much time training speakers to create syllables more efficiently.

We will attempt a definition here. In essence, a syllable may be defined as part of a series of motor speech movements involving successive openings and closures of the vocal tract and the consequent sounds those movements produce. This definition attempts to take the viewpoint of both speaker and listener, for both must be considered.

From the speaker standpoint, a syllable is considered here as a series of vocal tract movements, beginning with a relatively closed vocal tract posture, proceeding to a more open configuration, and returning to the relatively closed posture. A series of syllables is sometimes referred to as exemplifying running speech, and as these syllables flow, the open and closed postures usually differ in degree, depending upon the location and extent of vocal tract closure. Of course, a speaker can start with either an open posture or a closed posture and proceed to alternate opening and closure in some pattern assumed as the speaker wishes.

In any case, the simplest way to describe speech sounds in syllables is arguably by their degree of openness and closure. Jakobson (1968) theorized the possibility that one of the earliest distinctions a child learns in language development is the distinction between open and closed. Thus, the most open speech sound would be an open vowel, such as /ɑ/, while the most closed would be a plosive, such as /p/.

It is important to recognize that syllables most often occur in chains or series, over time, and that the closed vocal tract posture at the end of one may also serve the same purpose at the beginning of the following syllable. Articulation of syllabic boundaries requires the greatest precision of movement, and accuracy in articulating syllabic boundaries is most often a goal of speech therapy.

From the standpoint of the listener, a syllable can be considered as an acoustic impulse, of varying amplitude according to vocal tract patency or the degree to which it is unobstructed. In a manner similar to using a megaphone, the more open the vocal tract, the greater the acoustic energy amplitude.

THE PHONEME AND ARTICULATORY TARGETS

The concept of the phoneme and its allophones is sometimes difficult to grasp. Simply put, a phoneme is an idealized group of speech sounds produced with similar place, manner, and voicing characteristics that differentiate meaning by contrasting with other speech sound groups. Yet, no matter how hard a speaker may try, it is almost impossible to produce the same articulatory movements in exactly the same way over multiple trials, particularly when the differences result from the recent or upcoming articulation of previous or following speech. There will almost always be small differences, and these differences will produce slight acoustic differences in the sounds emanating from the vocal tract. The various speech sounds in a phoneme group with similar place, manner, and voicing characteristics are allophones of the phoneme group. These variations are not sufficient to change the meaning of the word in which they are used. The key to recognizing that a speech sound is an allophone of a phoneme is that the meaning of a word does not change when it is substituted for another allophone.

There are several key concepts to this definition. First is that a phoneme is a group of articulatory possibilities, each having a particular type of acoustic signal. Thus, it is impossible to utter a phoneme, since to do so would be to utter all the possibilities at once.

For example, variations within a plosive phoneme family might include the *release*, that action by which the impounded air is expelled. Two examples of plosive releases are *aspiration*, with audible noise emanating from the glottis, and *unreleased*, with no audible release. These represent two allophones of the phoneme /p/. Both are acoustically different, but is easy to see that both cannot be uttered simultaneously.

Another key concept in our phoneme definition is that phonemes underlie meaning in spoken language. It is not difficult to see that interchanging the above examples within a given word does not alter the semantic meaning of the word. /kæpʰ/ means the same as

/kæp ⌐/, even though there is an audible difference in the way the two utterances sound. At some point, though, the acoustic difference among the speech sound utterances becomes sufficient to cross over the phonemic boundary into another phoneme group, thus changing the meaning of the word. Perhaps those differences are enough to turn "cap" /kæp/ into "cat" /kæt/. When the acoustic differences in a vocal tract sound are sufficient to change meaning in the spoken language, the differences are termed *distinctive*, *contrastive*, or *phonemic*. By the way, changing a vocal utterance to make a meaningful word meaningless is making a distinctive difference, like substituting /p/ for /t/ in the word "bat."

Another interesting aspect of this meaningful concept is that if a sound produced by the vocal tract does not underlie some sort of meaning in a spoken language, it is not part of any phoneme group in that language. Thus, there are differences in the number of phonemes used to convey meaning in any language or, for that matter, in any dialect of any language. A vocal tract sound that does not underlie meaning is considered a *phone*. Thus, not all phones are allophones.

ARTICULATORY TARGETS

We have said that allophonic articulatory variations within a phoneme group do not change meanings in the words in which they are used, even though they sound slightly different. These acoustic differences can be seen on a speech spectrogram, yet these acoustic or articulatory differences are non-distinctive. They are produced at a given instant under conditions that are particular to that instant. It is very possible, even probable, that an individual speaker uttering the same series of syllables will generate another allophonic variation, different but not distinctive, in the next instant. The differences are subtle and most often dependent upon phonetic context, through the effects of variations in factors such as muscular effort, coordination, and inertia.

There is a range of acoustic and articulatory variation that is accepted within a phoneme group. Exceeding the perceptual boundaries of that range crosses the line into another phoneme group or category. This occurs when the listener perceives a meaning change in the utterance, and the line can vary among different listeners, according to a variety of factors particular to the listener, including, but not limited to, hearing acuity, listening ability, and linguistic background. The psycholinguistic function that listeners use to associate phonetic acoustics with phonemic meaning is called *categorical perception*.

Some have attributed allophonic pre-programming, that is, the tendency to pre-set the articulatory movements for a particular utterance, to a motor association function of Broca's area of the frontal lobe, but this is a very simplistic way to look at the process. There are many diverse and interconnected central nervous system inputs to the final common pathways for speech articulation (Lemaire et al., 2013). Linguistic learning is to some extent a function of brain plasticity, which, in turn, depends upon central nervous system development. Optimal development appears to depend on many factors, including sensorimotor experiences, socioeconomic status, parent and social relationships, pre- and post-natal events, diet, drugs, immune system status, and even intestinal bacteria (Kolb, Harker, & Gibb, 2017).

SYLLABLE BOUNDARIES AND SYLLABLE NUCLEI

The closed vocal tract postures assumed in syllable articulation are sometimes referred to as *syllable boundaries*, while the open vocal tract postures are called *syllable nuclei*. One might consider the flow of speech as opening and closing, with movements to and from the syllabic boundaries and nuclei. Syllable boundaries convey the major part of the linguistic information in syllables, while nuclei, by virtue of their more open postures, produce most of the acoustic energy. The combinations of closed boundaries and open nuclei produces variations in acoustic amplitude, creating the perception of acoustic pulsing for the listener.

Accuracy of articulation implies a target, and, indeed, articulatory targets are frequently described in classifying syllabic boundaries in terms of places of articulation. The concept of a target is appropriate in considering that a speaker aims to hit these places of articulation, but, like a marksman, may vary slightly in accuracy.

Places of articulation are described rather well by the IPA (2015) in terms of vocal tract structures brought into juxtaposition with one another. However, it must be remembered that so-called places of articulation specify only small parts of the vocal tract, and that the entire tract changes shape when the surfaces of its various parts are brought into juxtaposition. Speakers appear to preprogram articulatory targets, or idealized positions for phoneme articulation. In fact, the phoneme, itself, is an ideal; categorized as a group of articulatory possibilities with similar place, manner, and voicing characteristics; and expressed instantaneously as an allophone.

The concept of the articulatory target is furthered by the chart of the IPA, with its place of articulation nomenclature indicated as column headings in its pulmonic consonant chart. The IPA nomenclature is not entirely an accurate description of the articulatory process, since it tends to focus on a single or perhaps two articulators. We must remember that vocal tract configuration may be idealized by a speaker, or by the IPA, but the postures are formed by multiple muscular contractions and their effects on diffuse vocal tract regions, rather than by a few contractions at a specific site.

A very basic aspect of articulating syllabic boundaries is timing. The sequence of open-close-open-close-open… must be timed correctly for the speech to have its desired meaning. After all, articulating the second boundary in a syllabic chain may be recognized as either the end of the first syllable or the beginning of the second syllable. This is where the concept of juncture becomes relevant.

Simply put, syllable juncture is the manner in which syllables are connected in running speech. A more technically correct description would be the flow of movements in speech articulation. Juncture can be either open or closed. If syllabic juncture is closed, then there is no acoustically silent interval between syllables, and the boundaries of all but the first and last syllables are co-articulated. Most running speech is articulated with closed juncture. Speech articulated with open juncture can be said to be articulated one … syllable … at … a … time. There are clearly audible boundaries between syllables articulated with open juncture. It should be apparent that most speech is articulated with closed juncture, the usual exception being one-word utterances.

Syllabic boundaries have special significance to practitioners of speech-language therapy, for they are the most often encountered targets of treatment. Boundaries are almost always formed by pulmonic consonants or by blends of pulmonic consonants. Articulation of vocal tract structures produces changes in pulmonary air flow either by stopping the flow momentarily or by restricting it in conjunction with modification of vocal tract acoustic resonance. Even if a syllable is one that is usually considered to begin or end with a vowel, as written, the boundaries are, in fact, glottal consonants, as spoken.

If we consider that normal articulatory transition between syllables is closed juncture, it could be argued that most syllabic boundaries occur at the beginning of syllables, with articulatory postures moving from there toward and through the syllabic nucleus and on toward the next boundary. Because of the prevalence of closed juncture in normal speech, the speech therapist might consider concentrating on syllable onsets first, following up with intervocalic consonants between syllable nuclei, and turning finally to syllable arrestors, as needed.

The syllabic boundary that begins articulatory movements toward the syllabic nucleus is sometimes referred to as being in the *initial* position since, if the syllable were uttered without any other accompanying syllables, it would be the first posture assumed by a speaker. Imagine a speaker assuming a closed-lip posture just before producing the bilabial plosive that begins the word, "ball" (/bɑl/). This boundary is sometimes called a syllable releaser, or the syllable onset, since it is from this posture that the remainder of the syllable is formed. Implicit in this concept is the idea that a syllable is more than the sum of its boundaries and nucleus, but is, instead, a kinetic movement pattern. Note that it is impossible to utter /b/, or any other voiced plosive, without a following vowel. This principle of ongoing movement applies to running speech movements in general. Although it is possible to utter allophones in isolation, it does not occur very often. The first syllabic boundary is therefore also described as *pre-vocalic* with reference to its position before articulation of the nucleus, since syllabic nuclei are formed by *vocalic* phonemes: vowels, approximants, and nasals.

The opposite is the case for syllabic boundaries articulated after nuclei. These boundaries are said to be articulated in the *final* position, are syllabic *arresters* or *offsets*, and are *post-vocalic*. Since most syllabic transition is closed juncture, these final boundaries are articulated as such less often, since they arrest the flow of running speech. The final syllabic boundary, or offset, is also referred to as the *coda*, which is simply the Italian word for tail. The syllable nucleus, articulated with the coda, is sometimes called the *rime*. Note that syllables having the same nucleus and coda rhyme, such as "tail" /teɪl/ and "sail" /seɪl/.

The nucleus is the most open part of the syllable. It is usually a vowel or a diphthong, but can be a syllabic consonant. Syllabic consonants, you will recall, are nasals or approximants used to form syllabic nuclei. Their vocal tract postures are more open than obstruent consonants, and an old collective term for them is *semi-vowels.* The relatively open vocal tract posture of the nucleus produces the most acoustic energy in the syllable.

A syllabic nucleus may be *simple* or *complex.* A simple nucleus is a monophthong, with a single formant structure, while a complex nucleus might be a diphthong or even a triphthong, with formant ratios shifting through two or more patterns over time. The resonance of the nucleus also varies according to the posture of the coda, as the articulators move toward the next consonant target.

Although the syllabic nucleus, by virtue of its open articulatory posture, emits the most acoustic energy in speech, it is rarely the object of speech therapy treatment. This is probably because of the wider continuity of possible articulatory postures possible within a phonemically distinctive category, the relatively lower amount of linguistic information conveyed, and the wide variations acceptable in instances of lower syllabic stress and interspeaker variation.

This is not to say that vowels are inconsequential to syllable intelligibility; far from it. The reason for vowels being rarely targeted in speech therapy is that there is a wider range of acceptable variations in vowel articulation than in consonant articulation. Variations in tongue position create the vocal tract configurations necessary to achieve the required spectral characteristics, but among these, a certain amount overlap is permissible. Thus, articulatory precision is not as critical as it is for obstruent consonants or for approximants.

As far back as 1952, Peterson and Barney described the critical element for vowel identification as the relationship between the center frequencies of the first two formants. In a report that is still widely referenced today, they analyzed the spectrographic results of a group of 76 subjects articulating the words: heed, hid, head, had, hod (a tool for carrying bricks), hawed (past tense of hesitating utterance), hood, who'd, hud (the shell of a grain or nut), and heard. Some of these words seem archaic today, but they contain a wide range of vowels uttered as monosyllabic nuclei, and these nuclei are critical to their minimal pair intelligibility. The speakers uttered the target words from lists in which the words were arranged in random order, to reduce a practice effect, and each speaker read two lists.

The center frequencies of F1 and F2 were then plotted on a Cartesian coordinate system graph. The results showed considerable variation in F1/F2 ratios, which might be due to the effects of individual vocal tract dimensions, motor articulatory skills, and previous language experience. Today, we refer to these variations as

vowel space. There was overlap among vowels /ɛ, æ, ʊ, and ɝ/; among /ɑ and ɔ/; and among /ɝ and ʊ/, but other vowels were fairly well defined in terms of their spaces and, hence, distinction.

SYLLABLE TYPES

Syllables are often classified in terms of their boundaries, with the two main types being open and closed. An open syllable ends in a vowel, and a closed syllable ends in a consonant or consonant blend. Thus, the vocal tract might be considered as open at the end of articulation of an open syllable, and closed at the end of a closed syllable, with open syllables only articulated in the closed juncture circumstances of running speech.

A more detailed description of syllable types is provided by use of the letters C, to represent consonants, and V or N, to represent vowels or nuclei. The most popular designation of a syllable nucleus is V, but such designation is more of a tradition, since the nucleus of a syllable can be complex, as when a diphthong is present, or the nucleus can be a syllabic consonant, such as /m/, leading to the preference of an N (nucleus) as a more universal designation (see Figure 6.3-3).

By this method, an open syllable would be a CV, or CN, and a closed syllable would be a CVC or a CNC. Multiple abutting consonants, called blends, could be designated CC, etc., and affricates are designated with a single C.

"Buy" /baɪ/, for example, is an open syllable (CV or CN), as is "eye" /ʔaɪ/ (CV or CN), with the glottal plosive as the syllable releaser. "Sat" /sæt/ is a closed syllable, CVC or CNC, as is "flame" /fleɪm/, a CCVC or CCNC.

SYLLABIC STRESS

Syllabic stress, a suprasegmental feature of speech, imposes constraints concentrated primarily upon articulation of syllabic nuclei. Stressed syllables are articulated with more pulmonic and muscular pressure than unstressed syllables, creating more acoustic energy and more duration, so articulatory target acquisition is accordingly more precise. Syllabic stress is a relative phenomenon, such that syllables can be considered stressed only by comparison with other syllables uttered in the same context. This is the reason that it is never appropriate to transcribe a monosyllabic utterance with a schwa nucleus. Acoustic changes associated

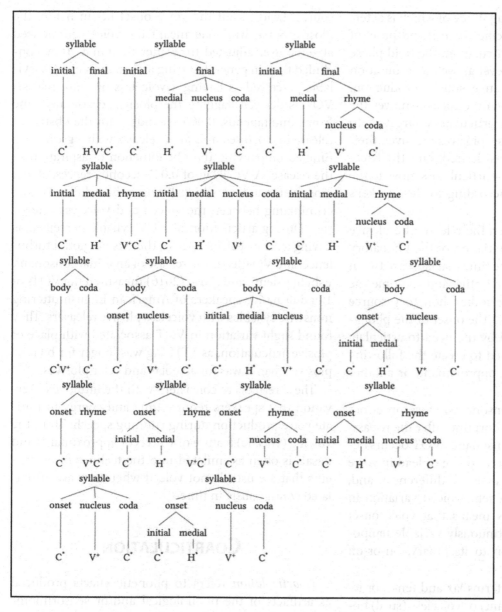

Figure 6.3-3. Descriptive syllable shapes and terms.

VOICE ONSET TIME

with stress have been well-documented. Fry (1955) found that duration and intensity ratios were critical values for stressed syllable perception with syllabic nuclei being more affected than syllable boundaries, while the work of Lehiste and Peterson (1958) found much the same but included a rise in fundamental frequency as an additional factor.

Although the phonatory source accompanies most speech, there are intervals during which the voice is not used, such as during articulations of unvoiced obstruent consonants and during pauses. Regarding the former condition, *voice onset time*, often abbreviated

VOT, is critical in the categorical discrimination between homophonous obstruent consonants. VOT is the temporal parameter marking the time that the phonatory source is initiated relative to the onset of the two other speech sound sources, the plosive and fricative sources. It is, thus, an important parameter by which listeners perceive distinctive differences in members of homophonous obstruent consonant pairs.

To properly appreciate VOT, one has to consider the phases of obstruent articulation: *foreglide*, *hold*, and *release*. During foreglide, the speech articulators move from their previous postures toward the place of articulation for the target obstruent. There is a brief hold phase, during which aerodynamic factors that create the plosive or fricative sources are created. For the plosives, a critical intraoral air pressure must be achieved during the hold phase, the magnitude of which is determined by the speaker for specific linguistic purposes of the moment. For fricative articulation, the hold phase requires a critical pressure level as well as a duration for speaker-determined fricative source production. The release phase occurs when the speaker moves the articulators toward the next articulatory target or to rest. During this release phase, plosives are given their various allophonic releases as desired, and the fricative source is suspended as the articulators move to the following phonemic target according to the speaker's desires.

VOT is the period between the release of a plosive or fricative source and the initiation of the phonatory source. In other words, it is the time that lapses between the release of a plosive or a fricative and the time the speaker initiates the quasiperiodic phonatory source (Abramson & Whalen, 2017). The onset of the phonatory source may be required by the need to articulate a voiced obstruent or the need to create the following phoneme, be it vowel, nasal, approximant, or another obstruent.

For voiceless, or surd, consonants, voice onset occurs simultaneous with or a short time after the release, while for voiced or sonant consonants, VOT occurs before the release. Varying degrees of lag or lead in voice onset time are perceived as dialectic differences, and, in some cases, distinguish a semi-voiced variation in non-English languages. This means that voice onset should be considered a continuously variable temporal phenomenon in addition to its binary, on-or-off characteristics.

Some linguists prefer the terms lax and tense, or lenis and fortis, to voiced (sonant) or voiceless (surd) homophone pairs. The distinction is based on the relative increase in muscular effort required to create the voiceless consonants than for the voiced consonants.

A problem with all these terms is that they only describe a subjective approach to homophone categorization and leave little objective basis for determining whether a consonant is voiced or not. A more objective determination can be expressed in the form of timing. A classic study by Lisker and Abramson (1964) attempted to define the differences between voiced and voiceless plosives with synthetic speech stimuli. The instruments generating these stimuli allowed the experimenters to manipulate VOT relative to the onset of a transient acoustic burst simulating a plosive source. Experimenters varied VOT from a lead of 0.150 seconds before, to a lag of 0.150 seconds after, the initiation of an artificial, electronically generated plosive

source. Lead meant the voice onset began before the plosive burst, while lag meant the voice commenced at some user-adjusted time after the burst. They concluded that, in general, during articulation of a CV syllable perceived as having a voiceless or tense release, VOT is delayed, lagging the plosive release any time from simultaneous, 0.000 seconds, with the obstruent release to 0.050 seconds after release, with a greater lag time accompanying the phenomenon of aspiration in the release. A VOT lag of 0.025 seconds represented a crossover point, at which listeners had difficulty discriminating between the voiced and voiceless categories. During articulation of a CV syllable perceived as having a lax or voiced release, there is no glottal turbulence, and VOT leads the release of an initial consonant. Eshghi, Alemi, and Zajac (2016) measured the VOTs of 10 adult native speakers of American English uttering nonsense syllables with voiceless plosive releasers. They found slight variation in VOT associated with place of plosive articulation, as VOT lag was longer for bilabial plosives than it was for alveolar and velar plosives.

These results are consistent with the intuitive observation that speakers require time and energy to initiate voice production during running speech. Thus, the voicing (vocalic) feature of vowels or approximants and nasals is often assimilated into the features of obstruents that are usually not voiced when they are articulated contiguously in time.

COARTICULATION

Coarticulation refers to phonetic effects produced as artifacts of the phonological and/or sensorimotor process of changing from one articulatory posture to another. A speaker can coarticulate phonetic segments consciously or unconsciously. Subject to phonetic context, the effects can be observed in anticipation of upcoming phoneme articulation through phonological processing, and in instantaneous articulation of a segment as a function of neuromuscular agility combined with the mass and momentum of the articulators (Tilsen et al., 2016). The very multitude of factors interplaying in coarticulation means that its effects are also highly individual.

The term coarticulation can also be taken to mean the simultaneous articulation of two phonemes. Notable examples of this are the English affricates /tʃ/ and /dʒ/. The /p/ and the /t/ in "optic" are often released simultaneously as a coarticulation.

Assimilation, the process by which features of one phoneme are carried over into articulation of another phoneme contiguous in time, is a type of coarticulation. It is, perhaps, most frequently observed when nasal consonants are articulated contiguously with vowels. This well-known condition results in *nasal assimilation* when vowels normally articulated with a predominantly oral resonance are articulated with nasal resonance. The normal speaker is simply unable to close the velopharyngeal sphincter fast enough to create a vowel with oral resonance immediately after uttering a nasal consonant, and particularly when the vowel is articulated between the articulation of two nasal consonants.

Assimilation can be progressive, regressive, or reciprocal. In progressive assimilation, sometimes called *left-to-right* assimilation, one or more features of a phoneme being articulated carried over to a following phoneme. The most frequently presented example of progressive assimilation is the common articulation of the word "captain" as "cap'n." In this example, the bilabial feature of /p/ is carried over in articulation of the upcoming syllable, eliminating its dental-alveolar-postalveolar releaser and vowel nucleus entirely and substituting a syllabic bilabial nasal for its arrester. Regressive assimilation is *right-to-left*. For example, the anticipated velar place of articulation in the second syllable releaser of income can change the place of articulation of the first syllable arrester from dental-alveolar-postalveolar to velar: /ɪnkʌm/ to /ɪŋkʌm/. Another commonly observed assimilation process occurs when two adjacent phonemes combine to form a third. Sometimes called *reciprocal* assimilation, an example occurs when /t/ combines with /j/ to produce /ʧ/, as when "Bet you" becomes /bɛʧə/.

Assimilation is a normal form of phonological processing, since it involves the influence that sounds and syllables have on each other when they are connected in the flow of speech. These influences result in phonetic changes brought about by the articulation or expectation of articulation of other phonemes.

Some forms of assimilation are so common that they are identified with special terms. *Epenthesis* occurs when a consonant is articulated as the result of the juxtaposition of two other consonants. A common example of this can occur when the nasal /m/ is followed by the fricative /θ/ in the word "something." An intrusive /p/ is created by the sudden release of air through the /m/ bilabial place of articulation when the velopharyngeal sphincter is closed to create sufficient intraoral air pressure for the upcoming dental fricative. The result is transcribed: /sʌmpθɪŋ/. Note that, in this

case, regressive nasal assimilation also occurs between the vowel nucleus and the nasal syllable arrester of the second syllable. One could argue that another extremely common example of epenthesis occurs when the English article "a" precedes a noun which is spelled with an initial vowel, changing "a" to "an." In epenthesis, the addition of a consonant is referred to as *excrescence*, while the addition of a vowel such as when /ʌ/ appears in that-a-way (/ðædəweɪ/) is called *anaptyxis*. Note that, in this example, the voicing feature of the intrusive vowel is regressively assimilated by the plosive between the first and second syllables.

The above examples of assimilation are independent of the semantic or syntactic linguistic structure of the utterance. In other words, a speaker can pronounce the above examples without the epenthetic consonant or vowel without changing the meaning or segmental sequencing.

Phonological processes such as assimilation can also be seen as a developmental phenomenon. Culbertson (2012) saw phonological development as a product of perceptual, neuromuscular, and anatomical maturation. As a child develops anatomically and physiologically, he or she will discover new articulatory possibilities, and, with proper nurturing, these will evolve into the phonology of the adult.

Assimilation processes are but one type of phonological process. Others include place or manner substitution processes and syllable structure processes. These processes are discovered in fairly predictable sequences through sensorimotor maturation processes, independent of their linguistic functions, and are explored and either adopted or extinguished, depending ultimately upon communicative value.

VELOPHARYNGEAL ARTICULATION

The velopharyngeal sphincter is a muscular valve situated between the nasopharynx and the oropharynx. The valve closes through elevation of the velum, commonly called the *soft palate*, by contractions of the levator velipalatini and tensor velipalatini muscles and, individually, by narrowing to varying extents the upper pharynx through contraction of the superior pharyngeal constrictor. This action disconnects or uncouples the nasopharynx form the vocal tract, creating a resonance described as oral. Opening the velopharyngeal sphincter couples the nasopharynx and nasal cavities with the vocal tract, creating a different shape and volume to the tube of the vocal tract, with distinct resonating characteristics described as nasal. In anatomical position, the force of gravity aids velar depression and nasal coupling, but the palatoglossus and palatopharyngeus muscles can act in support.

In addition to creating the necessary conditions for oral or nasal resonance, velopharyngeal sphincter closure must also be sufficient to allow intraoral air pressure to increase to the point that plosive and fricative sources can be created for obstruent consonant articulation. Complete velopharyngeal closure is not necessary, as some individual speakers can adapt to their individual anatomic and physiologic differences sufficiently to produce acceptable speech. Studies have shown that a velopharyngeal aperture of no more than 14 to 20 mm^2 is sufficient to allow creation of 294 Pa (reported as 3 cm H$_2$O) of intra-oral air pressure, judged as the minimum needed to produce plosive and fricative acoustic sources for the so-called *pressure consonants* (Dalston, Warren, Morr, & Smith, 1988), with the velopharyngeal sphincter requiring about 0.250 seconds of lead time to provide the desired vocal tract configuration (Bell-Berti, 1993).

A certain amount of nasal resonance is a desirable quality in the output spectrum of speech. The desired amount is variable, dependent upon the presence or absence of nasal phonemes in an utterance and listener preference. Too much nasal resonance in the output spectrum creates speech that is considered hypernasal, while too little nasal resonance is considered hyponasal. Fletcher (1974) developed a mask device to compare the amplitude of sound emanating from the nares with the amplitude of sound emanating from the combined oral and nasal openings, or total vocal tract. He designated this quantity nasalance, and apparently intended to market the device, the Tonar II, as a means of helping clinicians, researchers, and speakers to distinguish hypernasal and hyponasal speech from so-called normal speech. However, variation in listener appreciation and coarticulatory factors have made standardization of nasalance values elusive.

Agility in velopharyngeal sphincter action is also necessary for normal articulatory transitions. Individual differences in velopharyngeal sphincter function can affect speech to the extent that listeners attend more to the acoustic output than they do to the linguistic content. These differences can be the result of idiosyncrasy, congenital structural anomalies, central or peripheral nerve dysfunctions, disease, injury, or post-surgical conditions. The term *velopharyngeal inadequacy* describes the condition in which oropharyngeal and nasopharyngeal separation is ineffective in supporting distinctive oral or nasal speech, resulting in hypernasal speech.

Velopharyngeal inadequacy can be the result of velopharyngeal insufficiency or velopharyngeal incompetence. Velopharyngeal insufficiency can result from congenital conditions, such as maxillary clefts or of structural tissue changes following surgery, leaving the speaker with a lack of structural support for separation of the oropharynx and nasopharynx. On the other hand, in cases of velopharyngeal incompetence, there is sufficient tissue present to separate the cavities of the pharynx, but the speaker does not use the tissue adequately. Such a condition can be caused by paralysis of the velopharyngeal sphincter through central or peripheral nerve dysfunction. Alternately, the condition can be *idiopathic*, in which the cause of hypernasal speech is elusive, perhaps the result of atypical sensorimotor development, affective factors or learning.

Hyponasal speech is almost always the result of structural blockage of the nasopharynx or nasal cavity. A frequent and temporary cause is nasal blockage resulting from nasal inflammation or *rhinitis*. Another, more chronic cause of hyponasal speech is an abnormally large adenoid, or pharyngeal tonsil (Dworkin, Marunick, & Krouse, 2004).

Coarticulatory effects have led to the realization that velopharyngeal function in speech is more than a binary phenomenon. Bell-Berti (1993) reviewed research on the subject and reported several studies, some more than 100 years old, that supported the contention that velar height, hence degrees of velopharyngeal closure, was highly dependent upon phonetic context.

The distinctive resonating characteristics of nasal cavity coupling include attenuation of the overall acoustic output and the addition of antiresonances in the acoustic spectrum of the output (House, 1957). Antiresonances in the spectrum of nasal speech output dampen the formants present in the non-nasal (oral) wave and also add energy to low-amplitude frequency bands that are present, but not noticeable, in the non-nasal output spectrum.

Attenuation of the total acoustic output in nasal articulation is the result of the smaller dimensions of the nareal or nostril opening and the acoustic impedance created by nasal cavity tissues. Antiresonances are created by the presence of adjacent cavities along the direct vocal tract path. The nasal cavity is one of these adjacent resonant bodies, but others are created by varying volumes of the oral cavity. Oral cavity volumes, in turn, vary according to the particular nasal consonant's place of articulation. If the nasal consonant has a bilabial place of articulation, the volume of the adjacent cavity will be large, since the bilabial place is farthest from the pharynx. The alveolar nasal consonant will create a slightly smaller cavity, and the velar consonant will add the very smallest adjacent cavity volume to the vocal tract.

ARTICULATORY RATE

The rate of speech articulation depends on mass, range, flexibility, muscular opposition, and innervation of an individual's speech articulators, combined, of course, with maturation of the speaker's motor skills, personal intentions, the type of speech material (narrative, repeated, read aloud, and so on), and, perhaps, training.

A major influence on articulatory rate is *innervation ratio*, the comparison or ratio of the number of muscle fibers of a given muscle to the number of motor nerve fibers supplying the muscle. A high innervation ratio means there are many muscle fibers being served by few nerve fibers. This kind of ratio yields a strong but imprecise muscle. A low ratio muscle is weaker, but more precise. Among the speech articulators, the tongue is fastest, followed by the mandible. Interestingly, the lips are the slowest of the speech articulators.

Since the minimal motor unit of speech is the syllable, speaking rates might be best expressed as a rate of syllables per second. Tsao and Weismer (1997) reported the speech rates of 100 adults with presumably matured neuromuscular development in two groups: slow and fast speakers. The average rate for the slow group was 272.5 syllables per minute (standard deviation = 12.8), while the average rate for the fast group was 349.3 (standard deviation = 21.7). This worked out to 4.54 and 5.81 syllables per second, respectively. Standard deviation, a measure of variability, increased with rate in all groups. Redford's (2014) groups of 5- to 7-year-old children recorded articulatory rates somewhat slower than Tsao and Weismer's (1997) adults, ranging from 2.82 syllables per second for 5-year-old children to 3.84 syllables per second for 7-year-olds.

Tanner and Culbertson published the *Quick Assessment for Dysarthria* in 1999. The purpose of the assessment guide was to enable an evaluation of speech articulation, including speech rate, in a short time, so as not to spend an unnecessary amount of time evaluating, and spend more time stimulating patients in the early stages of recovery from a neurological insult. Thus, articulatory rates were to be assessed in

words-per-minute as either too slow or too fast. Words-per-minute are easier for a non-skilled practitioner to measure as a screening method when considering referral to a skilled speech-language pathologist. Optimal word-per-minute rates were judged to be between 136 and 204. A limitation of this approach, of course, is the fact that words vary widely in their number of syllables.

We have examined respiratory, phonatory, and oral-pharyngeal functions as separate entities, but only in the sense that each has certain attributes that bear closer study and play their own roles in the production of speech. It is clear that the vocal tract and the respiratory system must work effortlessly together to achieve normal speech. In this sense, they are the physiological effectors of speech.

REFERENCES

Abramson, A. S., & Whalen, D. H. (2017). Voice onset time at 50: Theoretical and practical issues in measuring voicing distinctions. *Journal of Phonetics, 63,* 75-86.

Bell-Berti, F. (1993). Understanding velic motor control. In S. R. Anderson, M. K. Huffman, R. A. Krakow, & P. A. Keating (Eds.), *Phonetics and Phonology, Volume 5, Nasals, Nasalization, and the Velum* (pp. 63-85). Amsterdam, The Netherlands: Elsevier. https://doi.org/10.1016/B978-0-12-360380-7.50007-7

Culbertson, W. R. (2012). Phonological processes and traditional phoneme acquisition norms. In Goldfarb, R. (Ed.), *Translational speech-language pathology and audiology: Essays in honor of Dr. Sadanand Singh.* San Diego: Plural.

Dalston, R. M., Warren, D. W., Morr, K. E., & Lynn, R. S. (1988). Intraoral air pressure and its relationship to velopharyngeal inadequacy. *Cleft Palate Journal, 25,* 210-219.

Dworkin, J. P., Marunick, M. T., & Krouse, J. H. (2004). Velopharyngeal dysfunction: Speech characteristics, variable etiology, evaluation techniques, and differential treatments. *Language, Speech and Hearing Services in Schools, 35,* 333-352.

Fletcher, S. G., Ph.D., Sooudi, I., & Frost, S. D. (1974). Quantitative and graphic analysis of prosthetic treatment for "nasalance" in speech. *The Journal of Prosthetic Dentistry, 32,* 284-291. https://doi.org/10.1016/0022-3913(74)90032-8

Fry, D. B. (1955). Duration and intensity as physical correlates of linguistic stress. *The Journal of the Acoustical Society of America, 27,* 756-768.

House, A. S. (1957). Analog studies of nasal consonants. *Journal of Speech and Hearing Disorders, 22,* 190-204.

International Phonetic Association (2015). Chart of the International Phonetic Association. https://www.internationalphoneticassociation.org/content/full-ipa-chart#ipachartkiel

Eshghi, M., Alemi, M., & Zajac, D. J. (2016). Aerodynamic and laryngeal characteristics of place-dependent voice onset time differences. *Folia Phoniatrica et Lopaedica, 68,* 239-246.

Jakobson, R. (1968). Child language, aphasia, and phonological universals. The Hague: Mouton.

Kolb, B., Harker, A., & Gibb, R. (2017). Principles of plasticity in the developing brain. *Developmental Medicine and Child Neurology, 59,* 1218-1223. doi:10.1111/dmcn.13546

Lehiste, I., & Peterson, G. E. (1958). Vowel amplitude and phonemic stress in American English. *The Journal of the Acoustical Society of America, 31,* 428-435.

Lemaire, J. J., Golby, A., Wells, W. M. 3rd, Pujol, S., Tie, Y., Rigolo, L., Kikinis, R. (2013) Extended Broca's area in the functional connectome of language in adults: combined cortical and subcortical single-subject analysis using fMRI and DTI tractography. *Brain Topography*, *26(3)*:428-41. doi: 10.1007/s10548-012-0257-7. Epub 2012 Sep 22.

Lisker, L., & Abramson, A. S. (1964). A cross-language study of voicing in initial stops: Acoustical measurements. *Word, 20*, 384-422. http://dx.doi.org/10.1080/00437956.1964.11659830

Peterson, G. E. & Barney, H. L. (1952). Control methods used in the study of vowels. *The Journal of the Acoustical Society of America, 24*, 175-184.

Redford, M. A. (2014). The perceived clarity of children's speech varies as a function of their default articulation rate. *The Journal of the Acoustical Society of America, 135*, 2952-2963.

Tanner, D. C., & Culbertson, W. R. (1999). Quick assessment for dysarthria. Oceanside, C.A.: Academic Communication Associates.

Tilsen, S., Spincemaille, P., Xu, B., Doerschuk, P., Luh, W., Wang, Y. (2016). Anticipatory posturing of the vocal tract reveals dissociation of speech movement plans from linguistic units. *PLoS ONE, 11 (1)*. http://dx.doi.org/10.1371/journal.pone.0146813

Tourville, J., Reilly, K., & Guenther, F. (2008). Neural mechanisms underlying auditory feedback control of speech. *NeuroImage, 39*, 1429-1443 doi: 10.1016/j.neuroimage.2007.09.054

Tsao, Y-C., & Weismer, G. (1997). Interspeaker variation in habitual speaking rate: Evidence for a neuromuscular component. *Journal of Speech and Hearing Research, 40*, 858-866.

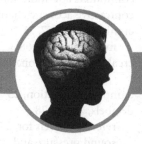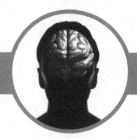

Index

abdominal pressure, 84
acceleration, 14
acoustic energy, 20
 amplitude of, 23–24, 74
 transforming into neurochemical potentials, 74
acoustic phonetics, 10
acoustic source, filtering, 38–39
acoustics, 10, 16
 basics of, 18–35
 vocal tract, 38
afferent impulses, 75
affricated release, 43–44
affricates, 43–44
allophone, 45
alveolar pressure, 84–86
amplitude, 23–24
 distance and, 29
 measurement of, 21
 in speech spectrography, 35
anaptyxis, 103
antiresonances, 43, 104
aphasia, 64
approximant articulation, 95
approximants, 42
apraxia, 60
Aristotle, 8
arrestors, 46
articulation
 feedback in, 94

muscle groups in, 94
speech sound sources in, 94–96
of syllables, 97
velopharyngeal, 103–104
articulatory muscles, 72
articulatory postures, 95
articulatory rate, 105
articulatory targets, 97–98
assimilation, 102–103
assimilation nasality, 43
associated structures, 69
association, 73
association centers, 69
auditory cortex, 76
auditory discrimination, 64
auditory pathways, 74
 central, 75–76
 synapses in, 76
auditory processing, 63–64
auditory system
 central, 75–76
 peripheral, 74–75
autonomic nervous system, 67

babbling, 51–52
bandwidth, 33
basal nuclei, 69
Bell, Alexander Graham, 24
Bernoulli, Daniel, 19, 83

Culbertson, W. R.
Fundamentals of the Speech and Language Sciences (pp 107-112).
© 2020 Taylor & Francis Group.

Bernoulli effect, 92
Blanc, Mel, 88
Boldrey, Edwin, 62
Boltzman, Ludwig, 11
Boyle's Law, 85
brain, 57, 66
    cerebral cortex of, 58–64
    cerebral dominance in, 64–65
    structure of, 58
    subcortical structures of, 65–66
brain stem, 66
breathing for speech, 82–83
breathy phonation, 88
Broca, Pierre Paul, 60
Broca's area, 55, 62
Brodmann, Korbinian, 58–59, 60, 61, 63
Brodmann's area, 62–63
Bruner, Jerome, 50
bucket handle movement, 85

categorical discrimination, 39–40
categorical perception, 98
centimeter-gram-second (CGS) system, 12
cerebellum, 66
    hemispheres of, 58
    in motor functions, 69
cerebral cortex
    areas of, 54–55
    frontal lobe of, 59–61
    functional centers of, 58–59
    motor functions of, 69
    occipital lobe of, 62–63
    parietal lobe of, 61–62
    temporal lobe of, 63–64
cerebral dominance, 64–65
cerebral hemispheres, 58
Clausius, Rudolph, 11
Clausius' Law, 11, 84, 85
clinical reports, language of, 6
clinical research, 4–5
closure, 73
coarticulation, 102–103
cochlea, 74–75
cognition process, 50–51
communication
    frontal lobe in, 59
    versus language, 50
complemental air, 82
complex waves, 30–31
conception process, 56
consonants
    approximant, 42
    nonpulmonic, 81
    obstruent, 43–44, 95–96
    pressure, 104
    pulmonic, 80–81

continuous aperiodic sound, 33
contrastive acoustic change, 40
cranial nerves, 67, 71
    motor fibers of, 68
creaky (pulsed) phonation, 88

dampened vibration, 25
decibels, 21, 24, 28
    reference levels for, 24–25, 28–29
    sound pressure and intensity and, 24
density, 15
    speed of sound and, 19
dependent variables, 4
Descartes, René, 26
diaphragm, 70, 85
diphthongs, 40
distance, 12
    measurement of, 13
    sound amplitude and, 29
distinctive acoustic change, 40
distinctive features, 46
distinctive resonance output, 40
driving source, 20, 38–40
dynamics, 9
dysfluent speech, 94

ear, anatomy and function of, 74
egressive speech sounds, 80–81
    muscles in, 70
eigenmodes, 92
elastic medium, 18
electric current, 12
electromagnetism, 8, 9, 11
energetic equilibrium, 11
energy fluctuations, 28
energy (work), 15–16
entropy, 11, 83
epenthesis, 103
equilibrium state, 20
experimental research, 4
expiratory reserve, 81, 82
extrapyramidal tracts, 69

facial muscles, 71, 72, 94
facial nerve, 71
falsetto phonation, 88
Fant, Gunnar, 41
feedback loop, 95
figure-ground discrimination, 64, 73
filter, 38–39
fluent speech, 94
force, 14
formant transitions, 43
formants, 35
formulation, 56
Fourier, Joseph, 33

frequency, 20–21, 35
Freud, Sigmund, 52
fricative sources, 38, 95
fricatives, 44, 96
  glottal, 88
  voiced, 35
functional transcranial Doppler measurement, 65
fundamental frequency, 31
fundamental quantities, 12–13

Galileo Galilei, 8, 9
gases, kinetic theory of, 19–20, 83–84
glottal flow waveforms, cycles of, 90
glottal postures, alternative, 87–88
glottal source, 39
glottal stop, 88
graphing spectra, 31–32
gravitation, 9, 10
gravity, 10, 12–13
gray matter, 58
gyrus (gyri), 58, 63, 76
  precentral and postcentral, 55, 69

hard palate, 94
harmonic frequencies, 31
harmonics of the fundamental, 31
heat, 12
Helmholtz resonator, 38, 41
  double, 39
Hertz, 22
Hertz, Heinrich, 22
Heschl's gyrus, 63, 76
homophone pairs, voiced or voiceless, 102
homunculus, 62
hypernasal speech, 43
hypoglossal nerve, 71, 72
hyponasal speech, 43, 104
hypothalamus, 58, 66
hypothesis testing, 2–3

imply/infer, 3
independent variables, 4
inertia, 9–10
inferential statistics, 3
infrasound, 23
ingressive air flow, 80
innervation ratio, 105
input spectra, 39
inspiration, 85
inspiratory reserve, 81, 82
integration, 73
intercostal muscles, 70, 85
International System of Units (SI), 12
inverse square law, 29

Joule, James Prescott, 15

kilograms, 13
kinematics, 9
kinetic energy, 11
knowledge, acquiring, 1–2

Ladefoged, Peter, 41, 42
language
  versus communication, 50
  phonemes and meaning in, 97–98
  phonology of, 44–46
  processing of, 76
  reception processes and, 56
  of research project, 6
  thought and, 50
language development, 51
  cognitive model of, 51–52
  learning model of, 52–53
  sociolinguistic model of, 53–54
laryngeal muscles, 71
laryngealization, 88
learning theories, 52–53
lemniscus, 76
length, 12, 13, 87
light, 12
linguistic milestones, 51–52
lip rounding, 41, 95, 96
listeners
  language processing in, 56
  thoughts in, 55
listening
  central auditory system in, 75–76
  peripheral auditory system in, 74–75
  stages of, 73
loudness, 21, 87
  amplitude and, 23–24
lung volume, 85
lungs, 80–82

mandibular elevation, 72
mass, 12
  versus force and weight, 14
  measurement of, 13
  in motion, 9–10
Maxwell, James, 11
meaning, phonemes and, 97–98
measurement systems, 12
mechanics, 9–10
medial geniculate body, 76
medium, 20
metalanguage, 51
meter, 13
meter-kilogram-second (MKS) system, 12
metric system, 12
modal voicing, 87–88
molecular quantity, 12
motion, Newton's laws of, 9

motor association area, 55
motor functions, voluntary and involuntary, 68
motor innervation, 54–55
motor speech functions, 68–69
motor speech processes, 93–94
movement, 9–10
muscles
    of speech, 69–72
    synergistic contraction of, 69
    types of, 68
myoelastic-aerodynamic principle, 91–92

nasal articulatory postures, 43
nasal assimilation, 102–103
nasal cavity, resonating characteristics of, 104
nasal consonant articulation, 43
nasal formants, 43
nasal murmur, 43
nasal resonance, 42–43, 104
nervous system, 57. *See also specific components of*
    central, 57–66
        motor speech functions of, 68–69
        speech muscles and, 69–72
    divisions of, 57
    peripheral, 57, 66–67
    speech muscles and, 69–72
neuroglia, 58
Newton, Isaac, 8, 9, 14
noise, 29
    definition of, 33
    narrow-band, 33
    signals and, 25
    wide-band, 33, 35
null hypothesis, 3

objects, 2
olivocochlear bundle, 76
open-closed concept, 45–46
optic nerve, 63
optic radiation, 62
oral cavity constriction, 40–41
oral cavity volume, 104
oral muscles, 71–72
output spectra, 39

parameters, 2
pars triangularis, 60
Pascal, Blaise, 14
Penfield, Wilder, 62
perception, 73
    categorical, 98
    occipital lobe in, 62–63
    of speech, 75
    temporal lobe in, 63–64
period, 20–21
periodic vibration, 22

peripheral nerves
    final common pathway of, 68
    injury to, 68–69
    motor fibers of, 68–69
phase, 29–30
phonation, 87–93
    closed phase of, 90–91
    myoelastic-aerodynamic principle of, 91–92
    open phase of, 91
    parameters of, 87
    viscoelastic aerodynamic theory of, 92
phonatory cycling, 90–93
phonatory durations, 87
phonatory frequency, 87
phonatory intensity, 87
phonatory muscles, 71, 94
phonatory source, 38, 87, 95
    quasi-periodic, 89
phonatory spectrum, 87
phoneme groups, 44–45
phonemes, 40
    articulatory targets and, 97–98
    oral muscles in producing, 71
    plosive, 43–44
    types of and vibration types, 23
phonemic acoustic change, 40
phones, 40, 44–45, 98
phonetic acoustic changes, 40
phonetics, 38
phonotactics, 46
physical science, basic concepts of, 7–8
physics
    classical, subdivisions of, 9–11
    modern *versus* classical, 8
Piaget, Jean, 51
pitch, 20–21, 87
place-manner-voicing, 46
pleural pressure, 84
plosive articulation, 33
plosive phoneme, 97
plosive source, 38, 95
plosives, 43–44
    glottal, 88
pneumatic power, 80
point of maximum constriction, 40–41
potential energy, 10–11
power, 15–16
power spectrum, 31–32, 33
pressure, 14–15
    changes in, 15
    study of, 10–11
psychological processes, 50
pulmonic air, cyclical valving of, 88
pulmonic speech sounds, 80–81
pulsation, 88
pump handle movement, 85

pure tone, 21, 22, 32
pyramidal tracts, 59–60

qualitative research, 4
quality, 87
quantitative research, 4, 7
quantity, 7, 11–12
    derived, 13–15
    fundamental, 12–13
quantum mechanics, 8
quantum physics, 11
quasi-experimental research, 4
Quick Assessment for Dysarthria, 105

R-blends, 42
reception, 73
reception processes, 56
referent, 52
relaxation pressure, 84–85
releaser, 45–46
research designs, 4–5
research hypothesis, 3
research papers, 5–6
research project, language of, 6
resonant vocal tract, 37–38
resonating cavities, 39
resonating systems, 38
respiration, physics of, 85
respiratory air flow, 85
respiratory cycles, 82
respiratory force balance, 86
respiratory muscles, 70–71, 94
respiratory pressures, 84
respiratory system in speech, 80–86
respiratory volumes, 81–82
running speech, 46–47, 95

scientific knowledge, 2
scientific method, 2
second, 13
semi-vowels, 42
sensation, 63
sensory homunculus, 61
sensory processing, 63–64
sequencing, 73
signal processing, 76
signal-to-noise ratio, 25, 29
simple harmonic motion (SHM), 25
    combining, 30–31
    graphing, 25–28
    phase and, 29–30
sine function, 26
sine wave, 26
sinusoidal curve, 26
sinusoidal wave, 27, 28
soft palate, 103

somesthetic cortex, 61
sound
    amplitude and distance of, 29
    definition of, 18
    inertia and gravitation in, 10
    intensity of, 28
        magnitude and, 23–24
        reference levels for, 24–25
    magnitude of, 23–25
    propagation of, 20
    sources of, 18
    speed of, 19
    vibrations and, 19–20
sound cycle, 25–28
sound energy, 20
    amount of, 28–29
    propagation of, 18–19
sound pressure, 20, 23
    level of, 24, 28
    magnitude and, 23–24
sound sources
    localization of, 74
    phonemes and, 40
sound spectrograph, 34
sound spectrum, 21, 30
sound wave propagation, 21
speech
    articulation and, 93–105
    breathing for, 82–83
    frontal lobe in, 60–61
    motor functions in, 68–69
    muscles of, 69–72
    neurological processes of, 50–56
    perception of, 75
    phonation in, 87–93
    processing of, 76
    respiration and, 80–86
    respiratory force balance in, 86
    spectrum of, 34
speech discrimination, 64
speech monitoring, 56
speech muscle groups, coordination of, 94
speech programming, 54–55
speech reception, 73
speech respiration, sustained gas flow in, 85
speech sound classification, 44–46
speech sound sources, 94–96
speech spectrography, 33–35
speed, 13–14
spinal cord, 57, 66
spinal nerves, 67, 68
spiral ganglion, 74
spirometer, 81
statics, 9
statistics, inferential, 3
steam power, 10

stereognosis, 62
striated (skeletal) muscle, 68–72
subcortical structures, 58, 76
subglottal pressure, 88–89
subvocalizations, 55
sulcus (sulci), 58
supplemental air, 82
surface, 13, 14
syllabic juncture, 46–47
syllabic stress, 100–101
syllable boundaries, 46–47, 98–100
syllable juncture, 99
syllable nuclei, 98, 99–100
syllables, 97
    shapes of, 101
    types of, 100
symbol, 52

temperature, study of, 10–11
thalamus, 58, 66, 76
Thales of Miletus, 8
theories, 2
thermodynamics, 8, 9, 10–11
    second law of, 84, 85
thorax
    expansion of, 70, 85
    recoil spring of, 86
thought
    frontal lobe in, 60
    in listener, 55
    neurological processes of, 50–51
tidal breathing, 82
tidal respiration, 85
tidal volume, 81–82
time, 12
    units of, 13
tongue muscles, 71
transient aperiodic energy, 33
transitions, 46
trigeminal nerve, 72
trigonometry, 26

ultrasound, 23
units, 12

variables, 2, 3–4
velocity, 13–14
velopharyngeal articulation, 103–104
velopharyngeal inadequacy, 104
velopharyngeal muscles, 71–72
vestibulocochlear nerve (cranial nerve VIII), 74–75
vibration
    amplitude of, 23–24
    aperiodic, 22, 23, 32–33
    dampened, 25
    descriptive terms of, 20–21

frequency of, 22–23
period of, 22–23
quasi-periodic, 22, 23
sound and, 19–20
timing parameters and patterns of, 20–23
vibratory cycle, 22
vibratory directions, 20
viscoelastic aerodynamic theory, 92
visual processing, 64
visual receptive centers, 62–63
vital capacity, 81
vocal folds
    adduction of, 88–89
    medial compression of, 88
    sounds produced by, 87–88
    vibratory characteristics of, 92
    vibratory frequency of, 91
vocal fry, 88
vocal tract, 37–38
    acoustics of, 38
    dynamics of, 46–47
    elastic medium of, 38
    resonating cavities of, 39
    sources of, 38
    structures of, 94
voice onset time, 101–102
voicing physiology, 88–89
volume, 15
    of resonating cavities, 39
    study of, 10–11
volume velocity, 90
vowel discrimination, 41–42
vowel identification, 100
vowel quadrilateral, 95
vowels, 40
    articulation of, 40–42
    back, 41
    central, 41
    front, 41
    vocal tract configurations of, 96
Vygotsky, Leo, 51

Wada test, 65
Watt, James, 16
weight, 12, 14
Wernicke, Karl, 54
Wernicke's area, 54, 62
whispering, 87–88
white matter, 58
Whorf. Benjamin, 51
Whorfian hypothesis, 51
wide-band noise, 33, 35
work (energy), 15–16
writing, 34

Zemlin, Willard, 64

Printed in the United States
by Baker & Taylor Publisher Services

Printed in the United States
by Baker & Taylor Publisher Services